healingstrong™

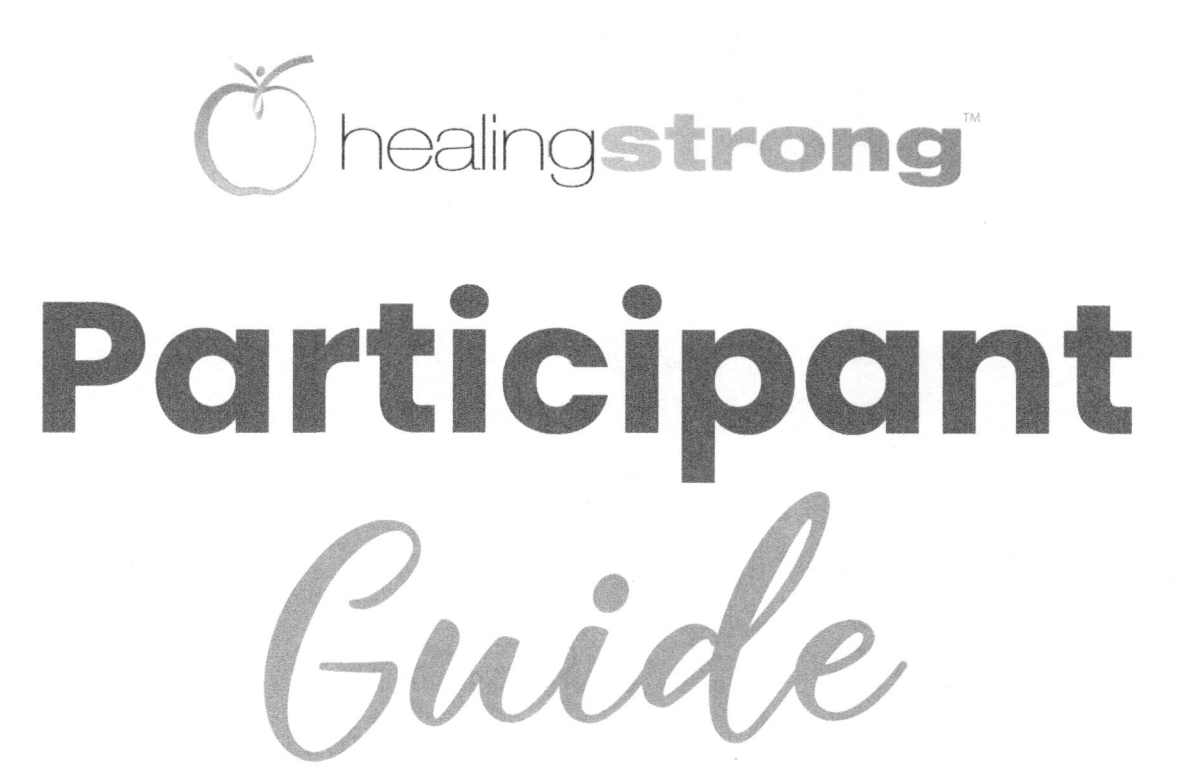

Participant Guide

Authors: Cortney Campbell and Suzy Griswold
Editors: Barbara Duck and Betty Roush (2023 Revision)

This guide is designed to accompany the lessons presented at your local HealingStrong™ group meetings. It includes a summary of each lesson presented by your HealingStrong™ group leader and all of the resources used in the lesson. It can also be used as a stand-alone resource even if you are unable to attend and makes an encouraging gift to a loved one who may have received a recent diagnosis. We hope you will find it incredibly helpful!

You can locate a local or online group near you by visiting our Groups page at https://healingstrong.org/group-directory.

Wisdom is the principal thing; therefore get wisdom: and with all thy getting get understanding.

Proverbs 4:7 (KJV)

Read or play before every HealingStrong meeting.

The content contained in these meetings are based on the HealingStrong™ "Group Leader's Guide & Curriculum", along with all other materials provided to you by HealingStrong™ which are not intended to be medical advice. The information is not intended to diagnose any medical or psychological condition, or to prevent, treat, or cure such medical or psychological conditions. The information is based on research conducted by the authors. HealingStrong™ encourages everyone to make their own health care decisions based on their own judgment, research, and experience. The information is not intended to replace a one-on-one relationship with a medical doctor or qualified healthcare provider. The Information has not been evaluated by the Food and Drug Administration nor the American Medical Association. Promotion of any and all products and services during this meeting is strictly for informational purposes only and not intended as an endorsement of such products or services. No goods or services are sold at these meetings. Guest speakers are not an endorsement by HealingStrong™ and agree also to adhere to the requirements of this disclaimer. HealingStrong™ reserves the right to use any photograph/video taken at this meeting. Although lessons are geared towards healing from cancer, these lessons are educational in nature and offer information that will equip and empower you with health choices and action steps that you can take that may benefit your overall well-being. If you are on a healing protocol, whether preventative in nature, or treatment that is conventional, holistic or integrative, the principles taught in these lessons may be applied towards a supportive plan for many health challenges. Thank you for joining us today!

From Our Hearts to Yours, Special Thanks

Thank you for taking this journey with our HealingStrong Community. Our intention is to equip you with a framework to help educate and encourage others. When there is a diagnosis of a serious illness, especially cancer, the thought of the disease and the treatment that follows many times, strips away dignity and hope.

We know this does not have to be! Knowledge empowers us to take control of our own health, operating in faith, and relinquishing fear. While you are encouraged to consult a licensed, qualified medical physician concerning your own or a loved one's health, you are also encouraged to be a well-informed self-advocate. In the end, the route one chooses to heal is an individual choice. HealingStrong™ does not ever want you to take our advice. Seek God first and His Wisdom. Learn the principles we teach because they are foundational principles that address healing the body and soul.

Our goal is to come along-side you to help educate, encourage and equip you with tools and strategies that will lead you into truth and wholeness. HealingStrong™ is a process, and while there are no guarantees on outcomes, by experiencing hope through implementing these strategies, connecting and encouraging in a group setting, one is empowered to own their own health. Healing requires big changes in one's lifestyle, including a shift in thinking and being intentional to connect with our Creator. It doesn't happen overnight, and there is not one way to heal that fits all. Hopefully, this curriculum helps you discover the basics.

While this guide addresses cancer head-on, the lessons support the wellness of individuals with any illness. Some may use this as a prevention tool, addressing barriers to a healthy, whole lifestyle. Take time to evaluate the information provided and apply it to yourself, and a group, whether it is a small gathering of friends, your family, or a larger community. The

The HealingStrong™ team has found we learn best from each other. The dialogue at our meetings is intended to be a two-way exchange. The personal connection we have at group meetings leaves us inspired and encouraged to continue. So, heal strong with a purpose. Share your story. Hope is needed.

HealingStrong™: Together, We Learn How!

God bless you and so much love,
Suzy Griswold & Cortney Campbell (Co-Authors)
Edited version by: Barbara Duck and Betty Roush, January 2023

HealingStrong™ Essentials

The HealingStrong™ Mission Statement:
Our mission is to connect, support, and educate individuals in community who are facing cancer and other diseases by focusing on strategies that help to rebuild the body, renew the soul and refresh the spirit through God's Word.

The HealingStrong™ Purpose:
To help others heal by creating a network of community groups online and in person that help to address the needs of body, soul, and spirit in order to find true healing and wholeness.

Three Pillars:
HealingStrong™ focuses on three pillars to accomplish its mission and purpose:

1) **Rebuilding the Body** - We support a growing network of online and in-person community groups with a curriculum that offers a holistic approach to wellness.
    a) By implementing the Anti-Cancer diet
    b) By practicing detoxification methods such as fasting and juicing
    c) By identifying and addressing nutrient deficiencies
    d) By gaining confidence through safe exercise
    e) By believing that God's design for healing also includes renewing your soul and refreshing your spirit
2) **Renewing the Soul** - We connect individuals to groups in their local area and online, who are learning to find hope and healing.
    a) By reframing our negative thought patterns
    b) By forgiving ourselves and others
    c) By practicing de-stressing techniques
    d) By incorporating gratitude into our daily routines
    e) By believing that God's design for healing also includes rebuilding the body and refreshing the spirit
3) **Refreshing the Spirit** - We offer faith-based encouragement through our many offerings on the Refresh page at https://healingstrong.org/refresh.
    a) By connecting with our Father in Heaven through community prayer and Bible study
    b) By learning to discern, hear and obey the voice of God
    c) By trusting God's promises found in His Word
    d) By discipling people into Truth
    e) By believing that God's design for healing also includes rebuilding the body and renewing the soul

Using the HealingStrong Lesson and Resource Guide

We hope this finds you well and eager to learn more about improving and taking charge of your health.

This guide is designed to accompany the lessons presented at your local HealingStrong™ group meetings. It includes a summary of each lesson presented by your HealingStrong™ group leader and all of the resources used in the lesson. It can also be used as a stand-alone resource even if you are unable to attend and makes an encouraging gift to a loved one who may have received a recent diagnosis. We hope you will find it incredibly helpful!

You can locate a group near you by visiting our Groups page at https://healingstrong.org/-group-directory. Online groups are also available to join.

This guide will give you an idea for many of the topics we discuss at our meetings and an abundant amount of resources to dig into learning more about the topics discussed.

Please note that although you will hear some of our lessons addressing the healing of cancer, the strategies recommended are helpful in improving many other health challenges as well. We are happy you are here!

Blessings on your healing journey! The HealingStrong™ Team

A Note About our FIYAA Affirmation Handouts:

At the end of each HealingStrong™ meeting we are reminded of how essential the right attitude is for healing. Through our FIYAA affirmation we affirm we will:

1. **F**orgive myself and others.
2. **I**nvite God into all aspects of my life and healing.
3. **Y**ield to the needs of my body during this healing season.
4. **A**ccept my diagnosis and symptoms as temporary.
5. **A**bandon negative expectations and think POSSIBILITIES!

Many HealingStrong™ participants choose to make copies to cut out and place throughout their home, car, and workplace as reminders. We've included a card below for you to share and copy as needed.

Also, don't forget that after each lesson you will find a recommended recipe to try and a scripture card for encouragement throughout your day. Feel free to share!

FIYAA AFFIRMATIONS

I will:

- **Forgive** myself and others.
- **Invite** God into all aspects of my life and healing.
- **Yield** to the needs of my body during this healing season.
- **Accept** my diagnosis and symptoms as temporary.
- **Abandon** negative expectations and think possibilities.

WWW.HEALINGSTRONG.ORG

Lesson 1:
Introductory Group Lesson

> **NOTE:** The full Participant Guide is available for download at our Start Here Page https://healingstrong.org/start-here. Please also review our full disclaimer for HealingStrong™ at: https://healingstrong.org/start-here.

My HealingStrong™ Group Information

GROUP LEADER: _____

CONTACT INFO: _____

MEETING LOCATION: _____

MEETING DATE/TIME: _____

OTHER INFO: _____

_____

_____

_____

_____

_____

Lesson Objective & Key Concepts

Take Away/Objective:
Participants will have an opportunity to meet one another, get to know the group leader and his/her connection to natural strategies, and understand the layout for the next 12 lessons including what will be covered.

Key Concepts:

- The HealingStrong™ Group is a local, independent group of patient-to-patient advocates and educators who desire to help others to heal strong and stay strong using natural strategies.

- The HealingStrong™ Group will follow a 12-month curriculum that will follow lessons created by HealingStrong™ that will introduce principles of diet, detoxification, exercise, emotional healing, non-toxic protocols and adjunct therapies, and each meeting will be launched with promises based on the very word of God.

- HealingStrong™ does not provide medical advice, and never sells goods or services at any of our meetings.

- HealingStrong™ Groups are about connections and authenticity where people come who desire to learn more about natural strategies, and seek to share their own experiences for the sole purpose of encouragement, education, and support.

- HealingStrong™ is supported primarily by volunteer efforts and donations from within the community. We are not persuaded by industry and therefore rely on our community for support. If you are interested in learning more about HealingStrong™, please go to the HealingStrong™ website: http://healingstrong.org.

Discussion Points

***Note to the Reader:** Although lessons are geared towards healing from cancer, these lessons are educational in nature and offer information that will equip and empower you with health choices and action steps that you can take that may benefit your overall well-being. If you are on a healing protocol, whether preventative in nature, or treatment that is conventional, holistic or integrative, the principles taught in these lessons may be applied towards a supportive plan for many health challenges.

The HealingStrong™ Mission Statement:
Our mission is to connect, support, and educate individuals facing cancer and other diseases through strategies that help to rebuild the body, renew the soul and refresh the spirit through God's Word.

The HealingStrong™ Purpose:
To help others heal by creating a network of community groups online and in person that help to address the needs of body, soul, and spirit in order to find true healing and wholeness.

HealingStrong™ focuses on three pillars to accomplish its mission and purpose:

Rebuilding the Body:

By implementing the Anti-Cancer diet

By practicing detoxification methods such as fasting and juicing

By identifying and addressing nutrient deficiencies

By gaining confidence through safe exercise

By believing that God's design for healing also includes renewing your soul and refreshing your spirit

Renewing the Soul:

By reframing our negative thought patterns

By forgiving ourselves and others

By practicing de-stressing techniques

By incorporating gratitude into our daily routines

By believing that God's design for healing also includes rebuilding the body and refreshing the spirit

Refreshing the Spirit:

By connecting with our Father in Heaven through community prayer and Bible study

By learning to discern, hear and obey the voice of God

By trusting God's promises found in His Word

By discipling people into Truth

By believing that God's design for healing also includes rebuilding the body and renewing the soul

All of our lessons center on helping an individual to obtain optimal health and well-being through the content and exercises that we will discuss. We will also provide resources at the end of a lesson or section that we will share with you for further study.

OUR LESSONS

Each meeting will provide an opportunity for you to be introduced to a strategy that we believe is important to living in full health. All of our lessons are research-based and evidence driven. Follow up resources will also be provided, along with a recipe and affirmation/prayer handouts that you can take home with you. The information in the lessons will align with the HealingStrong™ purpose.

Our lessons will cover the following topics:

- Taking charge of our health
- Cancer basics and first steps towards healing
- Helpful supplements and what NOT to eat during healing
- Seven steps for choosing a non-toxic cancer protocol
- Healing protocols and adjunct therapies
- Basics on toxins and why we need to detox to heal
- Strategies to detox
- Emotional healing
- Exercise
- Dental toxins and their impact on your health
- Sleep, meditation and breathing

Become a Supporter:

HealingStrong™ is supported primarily by volunteer efforts and donations from within the community. We are not persuaded by industry and therefore rely on our community for support. If you are interested in learning more about HealingStrong™, please go to the HealingStrong™ website: http://healingstrong.org.

Because of generosity, thousands of people each month know that there is a place that they can come to that offers hope, no matter the prognosis. We believe that together, we can heal stronger, and your help makes all the difference. If you would like to become a supporter, please go to our website: https://healingstrong.org/donate.

EMPOWER: Affirmations/Prayers

At the end of each lesson you will find a list of resources as well as a recipe, an affirmation, and a prayer. Furthermore, after each lesson we will read the HealingStrong™ FIYAA Affirmation for our overall healing. (See below in the CONNECT section).

We recommend that you connect with HealingStrong™ via the following:
HealingStrong™ Website: http://healingstrong.org/resources
HealingStrong™ Facebook page: http://www.facebook.com/healingstrong/
HealingStrong™ Instagram page: https://www.instagram.com/healingstrongofficial/

Good, Better, Best Tips

Introduction for section on Good Better Best:
As each lesson concludes, we want to leave you with an idea(s) for how to implement a suggestion from the lesson in an incremental fashion that meets your needs and abilities. Each lesson will give you ideas that are "Good, Better, and Best".

Good Tips: A perfect way to get started implementing healthier healing options. This tip will be less involved from both a time, energy, effort and financial resources.

Better Tips: This tip will progress you further into implementing the lesson idea. More time and cost may be involved in this step.

Best Tips: When you are ready, this tip will give you ideas to help implement the lesson ideas in a more extensive fashion. This could mean significant investment of time, energy, effort, and financial resources.

LESSON 1:

We Heal Better In Community!
Did you know that social support has a dramatic impact on our overall well-being. (See https://www.ncbi.nlm.nih.gov/pmc/articles/PMC2921311/)

Good: Make sure you have a friend(s) or family member(s) you can call on, who understands your choices for healing, believes in you, and will encourage you to keep moving forward along your path.

Better: The HealingStrong™ on-line community can offer support, education and encouragement. Review our site and see all it has to offer for support. https://healingstrong.org

Best: Join a local HealingStrong in-person or on-line community so that you can get to know local folks walking through a similar journey, or who have experience with it. Exchange phone numbers, meetup for lunch or a cup of tea, but connect! If you don't have one in your community, consider starting a group! https://healingstrong.org

Discussion Questions/Action Steps:

1. Congratulations for taking the first step and attending this HealingStrong™ meeting. What areas are you most excited to learn about?

   _____
   _____
   _____
   _____
   _____

2. What have you already done to begin your HealingStrong™ journey?

   _____
   _____
   _____
   _____
   _____

3. Do you have someone in mind that would help provide you support and accountability along the way (possibly joining in on group meetings)? If so, who is that person?

   _____
   _____
   _____
   _____
   _____

4. How will you stay engaged and focused this month on keeping your health a priority?

   _____
   _____
   _____
   _____
   _____

CONNECT:

As a participant in a HealingStrong™ group, you have much to take advantage of in your healing journey. Our meetings are just a part of helping you on a consistent basis. Review these resources for things that can help Rebuild, Renew, and Refresh you all month long!

HealingStrong™ website: http://healingstrong.org
HealingStrong™ Facebook page: http://www.facebook.com/healingstrong/
HealingStrong™ Instagram page: https://www.instagram.com/healingstrongofficial/
HealingStrong™ I AM HealingStrong™ Podcast page: https://healingstrong.org/podcast
HealingStrong™ Start Here: https://healingstrong.org/start-here

Remember: "Fear is detrimental to healing, but affirmations based on God's Word help us replace it with courage and strength."

FIYAA AFFIRMATIONS

I will:

- **Forgive** myself and others.
- **Invite** God into all aspects of my life and healing.
- **Yield** to the needs of my body during this healing season.
- **Accept** my diagnosis and symptoms as temporary.
- **Abandon** negative expectations and think possibilities.

WWW.HEALINGSTRONG.ORG

Being a faith-based organization, we are not only passionate about your present healing journey, but also passionate about your eternal destiny as well. Of course, there will come an end to this life for all of us. We want to make sure that we have shared with you how to know that your eternal destiny is in heaven with our Creator, the One who formed you, loves you, and made a simple way for you to know for certain. If you are not a believer in Jesus Christ and would like to learn more about His saving grace, please see these resources: https://healingstrong.org/refresh

NOTES

Lesson 1 Additional Resources for Further Use

Review the HealingStrong™ webpage: http://healingstrong.org If you are not already signed up for the newsletter, please do. We send out a handful of emails each month featuring more stories and resources for HealingStrong™.

Begin your journey by reviewing the resources available at: http://healingstrong.org/resources.

If you would like a participant guide for your own personal study, please download yours at:

http://healingstrong.org/resources. You may also order a copy from Amazon or your HealingStrong™ leader may have purchased copies for distribution.

Video of "why do groups matter?" https://player.vimeo.com/video/233323781
HealingStrong™ Conference, Atlanta, GA

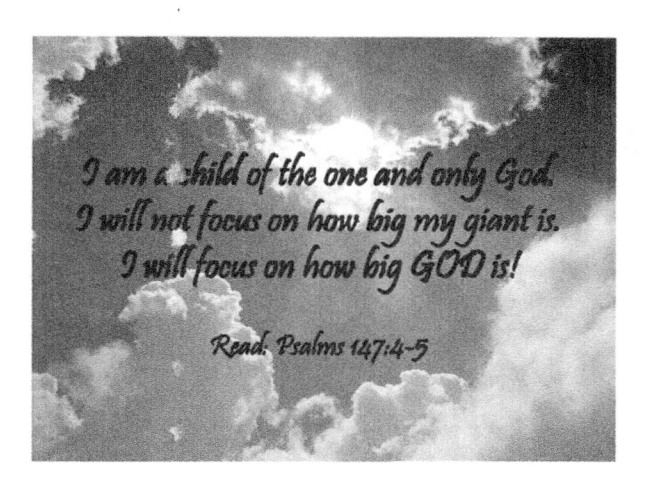

I am a child of the one and only God.
I will not focus on how big my giant is.
I will focus on how big GOD is!

Read: Psalms 147:4-5

Your Word says:

Turn, O Lord, and deliver me; save me because of Your unfailing love.
Psalm 6:4 NIV

Father God,

I come to You today searching for answers, comfort, peace and Your unfailing love for me. I know that You are the great healer and that all things happen according to Your divine plan. I know that Your love is greater than any struggle I face. Please help me and my family to feel the blessing of Your love no matter what. I pray that Your warriors surround and support every aspect of my life. When I am weary, Your love carries me. When I am uncertain, through medical guidance and advisors, Your path be declared. In Jesus' name I pray. Amen.

The Lord your God is with you,
the Mighty Warrior who saves.
He will take great delight in you;
in his love he will no longer rebuke you,
but will rejoice over you with singing. - **Zephaniah 3:17**
NIV
Thank you for the promises in YOUR Word. Amen.

Kale Salad with Walnuts and Mandarins
by Sandra Campbell

- 1 bunch kale, washed and torn into small pieces
- Himalayan sea salt
- 1 lemon, juiced
- 1 avocado

Walnuts, rough chop (can use cashews, almonds, etc. – your choice) 2 mandarin oranges (can use cuties), peeled and sectioned (can use pears or apples also).

Massage kale with a little salt – add lemon juice and continue massaging – then add avocado and mash everything together well – Put in a serving bowl and sprinkle on walnuts and mandarin orange sections. It keeps well for a couple of days in the fridge.

Good source of vitamins A, C, K and B6. Contains calcium, potassium, copper, manganese, protein, thiamin, riboflavin, magnesium, phosphorus and folate. Supplies protein and dietary fiber.

Lesson 2:
Building Confidence: Your Right to Take Charge of Your Health

> **NOTE:** The full Participant Guide is available for download at our Start Here Page https://healingstrong.org/start-here. Please also review our full disclaimer for HealingStrong™ at: https://healingstrong.org/start-here.

LESSON OBJECTIVES & KEY CONCEPTS

Take Away/Objective:
A person's ATTITUDE and THINKING make the biggest difference in overcoming the challenges that come with a cancer diagnosis or health challenge and choosing holistically-minded care.

Key Concepts:

- Cancer is survivable, and tumors are the body's natural defense to better manage and control the cancer development.
- Your positive or negative beliefs about your condition influence your body's response to healing.
- Educating yourself about your disease's behavior and choice of healing protocol is important to the success of your healing.
- Learning how to advocate for yourself and finding a doctor who works alongside you greatly increases your confidence.
- You do not owe anyone an explanation for your choice of healing strategy. You will learn how to respond to well-meaning friends and relatives' concerns and advice.

DISCUSSION POINTS

***Note to the Reader: Although lessons are geared towards healing from cancer, these lessons are educational in nature and offer information that will equip and empower you with health choices and action steps that you can take that may benefit your overall well-being. If you are on a healing protocol, whether preventative in nature, or treatment that is conventional, holistic or integrative, the principles taught in these lessons may be applied towards a supportive plan for many health challenges.

Cancer is Survivable and Healing is Possible

Introduction: It is so important to remember that we are all on a healing journey, one that is life-long. To view healing from cancer or any chronic disease as a destination is to set yourself up for possible burnout and defeat. The holistic and alternative path is certainly one less traveled and may feel lonely at times, hence the purpose of HealingStrong™ Groups. Both the physical and emotional aspects of healing can be challenging. Much of your insight and empowerment will come in discussion with others, which is why lessons are intended to be interactive. Please feel free to take notes and ask questions. We highlight cancer in this chapter; however, these principles apply for any chronic condition or disease.

- Your belief about cancer or any other disease will greatly impact your attitude on a healing journey.
- Healing with the whole body in mind is not just about dietary changes. You need to pay careful attention to thought processes and messages you send to yourself as well. Cancer is not some foreign invader that has come to take over your inner terrain.
- You can find lots of survivor stories that use natural healing. Here are a few sites that offer inspiration:
    - https://healingstrong.org/rebuild
    - http://www.radicalremission.com/index.php/blog
    - http://www.chrisbeatcancer.com/category/natural-survivor-stories/
    - https://cancercompassalternateroute.com/testimonials/
    - https://templetonwellness.com/cancer-survivor-stories/
- Pay careful attention to your thought processes and messages you send to yourself.
- See cancer as a wake-up call to make the changes the body and mind are craving.
- Believing this information about the body's ability to heal itself will greatly increase confidence in choosing a natural route to healing and visualizing it taking place.
- Cancer is a Preventable Disease that Requires Major Lifestyle Change. https://www.ncbi.nlm.nih.gov/pmc/articles/PMC2515569/
- Review this article that discusses "Cancer Is Not a Disease - It's a Survival Mechanism (Book Excerpt)." http://www.naturalnews.com/022578_cancer_body_disease.html

- Some resources that may be helpful:
  - Brenda Stockdale's book, *You Can Beat the Odds*
  - Dr. Caroline Leaf's book, *Switch On Your Brain: The Key to Peak Happiness, Thinking, and Health*
  - Mark Rutland's book, *Courage to Be Healed: Finding Hope to Restore Your Soul*

Finding Healing Confidence
- Be empowered to take charge of your health and get the care you desire.
- For some of you, optimism and confidence comes naturally. You have always questioned your doctor's medical advice, depending on your own research and intuition when it comes to your health care. Others of you may not like challenging the norm and find yourselves uncomfortable asking the difficult questions that come with choosing a more natural or holistic healing route. Many of you will be somewhere in-between, depending on the moment.
- You should feel empowered and peaceful in taking charge of your health and getting the care you desire, not simply defaulting to your doctor's choice because of fear of asking for what YOU need. Remember that YOU hire your doctor to work alongside you.
- Believe that what you are using to treat your cancer is the best choice for your healing and will WORK.
- See 5 Tips for Cancer Confidence by the Anti-Cancer Mom: http://www.anti-cancermom.com/a-day-in-the-life-5-tips-for-cancer-confidence/

Thoughts and Words Matter
- ATTITUDE and THINKING have an impact on your health.
- Pay attention to your body and how it FEELS different when you think in a positive, truthful way versus a negative, defeating way.
- Constant reinforcement in BELIEVING you will heal and are on your way to making permanent changes will help.
- Many times, old patterns of thinking resurface even after practice.
- Negative thought patterns often reflect our "core" beliefs about ourselves and God.
- Train your brain to notice negative thoughts and replace them with positive, truthful ones.

EXAMPLE:

Negative ⇨	I might not heal if I go against what my doctor says. I wish I had control.
Negative ⇨	I knew I was going to get sick. So many in my family have this same disease.
Negative ⇨	I don't have the willpower to do what it takes to make the changes I need to make.
Positive/Renewed thought ⇨	Getting sick is a wake-up call, and I need to treat my body differently. It's time to take care of myself.
Positive/Renewed thought ⇨	This disease is not a foreign invader but my body's way of telling me an imbalance needs to be corrected.
Positive/Renewed thought ⇨	Learning how to be kind to my body by giving it the right nutrition, detoxing it from the bad stuff I've been giving it all these years, and learning how to let go of negative emotions are ways that will support my healing.
Positive/Renewed thought ⇨	There are so many positive things I can do to contribute to my optimal health. God made my body and I can learn to take care of it properly.

- This thought passes in the blink of an eye. It is even more of a feeling than it is an actual dialogue in your head. You will feel its power over you. Your neck or back muscles tense. You feel sick to your stomach. You feel sad and anxious. These types of thoughts represent lies that are barriers to true healing.
- However, your thoughts have real power. Substitute a defeatist thought and the accompanying stressful, alarming, biological response with an empowering thought that brings increased peace and focus.
- As you shift your mindset and mental dialogue, pay attention to how your body feels in your chest, shoulders, and neck.
- Sometimes it takes repeating or even writing your renewed thought on a sticky note and re-reading it to help you believe it. When your mind considers it a truthful option, your body believes it too and responds accordingly. Your body really was designed to live in health! You can heal! *"Do not conform to the pattern of this world, but be transformed by the renewing of your mind. Then you will be able to test and approve what God's will is—his good, pleasing and perfect will." Romans 12:2 (NIV)*
- One resource to use is Fast from Wrong Thinking on the Bible app: https://www.bible.com/reading-plans/13766-fast-from-wrong-thinking

Become An Expert On The Disease's Behavior

- Use your oncologist or specialist to help you learn about how your cancer or disease behaves.
- The recommended treatment plan is just that: a recommendation. It is your body and your decision.
- Holistic minded medical doctors, naturopaths, and chiropractors can also share insight and direct you to options that a conventional doctor's office doesn't typically offer as a standard of care.
- Testing is a great way to understand your cancer better. Here are some resources to review as options:

- - HealingStrong's™ Healing Journey Jumpstart video on "How to measure and track your progress through testing: https://vimeo.com/662119052/4d405ee884
  - https://gcmaf.se/patient-resources/nagalase-blood-test/
  - https://www.rgcc-group.com/tests/
- Download and review Chris Wark's 20 Questions for Your Oncologist, at: https://healingstrong.org/resources

EXAMPLE:

If you are a cancer patient, understanding the following will help you will help you speak intelligently about your healing choices and ask further questions for clarity:
- how a tumor or cancer acts: https://www.cancer.gov/about-cancer/understanding/what-is-cancer
- It's typical rate of growth
- how it progresses
- what the "standard of care" is

THINGS TO CONSIDER WITH YOUR MEDICAL PRACTITIONER:

- Ask for a copy of every test and report.
- Make sure you have access to your results through any online portal available.
- Ask to look at the drug information inserts – the actual pharmaceutical inserts – that come with the recommended therapies.
- Keep a binder or online record of all of the handouts you receive and take notice of how many of them actually teach you how to help your body repair itself and heal – not many.
- If you would like to record a session with your doctor to later recall important information, it is advised to ask permission first (recording without permission may not be legal in your area).
- If you are being asked to come into a meeting with your doctor alone and are concerned with this, then ensure you take someone with you. You may tell them that because of your diagnosis, you need an advocate with you and that advocate is your loved one or friend. Or you may tell them you do not feel adequately prepared to take the notes and make decisions without a loved one. You may also tell your doctor that you are having trouble remembering things. If they are still giving you a difficult time, consider a new doctor.
- Ask questions like: What are the chances the treatment will CURE me? What are the long term effects of the treatment?

Find a Supportive and Cooperative Doctor
- Decide if your doctor is the right doctor to support your healing choice.
- If not, make it clear that you are not interested in the treatment plan, and ask if you can be monitored.
- This person should be there to work beside you, rather than try to convince you to change your mind, talk to you in a condescending way, or leave you feeling scared and discouraged (remember, negative thoughts and feelings affect your progress).
- You may find the right fit in a naturopath, homeopath, or holistic MD rather than a conventional oncologist or medical doctor.
- Your doctor is YOUR CHOICE. It is okay to find another who better fits your needs.
- Here are some support resources for your journey:
  - Square One - Coaching Course - Chris Beat Cancer https://healing-strong.org/resources
  - Breast Cancer Conqueror Coaching Program http://breastcancerconqueror.com/coaching/

Handling Concerned Loved Ones
- You do not owe anyone an explanation for your choice of healing strategy.
- While you are healing is not the time to explain why you are choosing an integrative or holistic route, especially to naysayers. Your journey and choice to heal in a manner that may be less conventional may offend some, and they may want to debate you, or criticize you. This is not the time to take that on. It is important to seek wisdom and understanding and preserve sound judgment and discretion. There is a nugget of truth in this verse: *"Do not give dogs what is sacred; do not throw your pearls to pigs. If you do, they may trample them under their feet, and turn and tear you to pieces."* Matthew 7:6, (NIV)
- This is a season where people that don't support you need to be kept at a distance.
- Set boundaries, being clear that you respect others opinion, but it's just that: THEIRS.
- Consider starting a web page (i.e: Facebook page devoted to updates, or a Caring Bridge page) where you can offer mass updates if you are comfortable.
  - Disable the comments so no one can offer an opinion.
  - Be clear that you ask for only positive and encouraging messages or emails. You do not owe anyone an explanation.
  - Be very cautious on using your personal social media page as a way to keep people informed. You will end up managing comments and going back to it over and over again. This is a time to keep off social media and keep focused on God's Word and your healing plan.
- Make sure your choice of treatment is part of a prayerful and well-researched process. Seek wisdom but gain understanding. See Proverbs 4:5-9 (NIV)
- Read, watch, and listen to the resources in this lesson.
- Take time to get quiet in the presence of God.

"Make me know Your ways, Lord Teach me Your paths. Lead me in Your truth and teach me, For You are the God of my salvation; For You I wait all the day."
Ps. 25:4-5 (NASB)

Good, Better, Best TIPS

Introduction for section on Good Better Best:

As each lesson concludes, we want to leave you with an idea(s) for how to implement a suggestion from the lesson in an incremental fashion that meets your needs and abilities. Each lesson will give you ideas that are "Good, Better, and Best".

Good Tips: A perfect way to get started implementing healthier healing options. This tip will be less involved from both a time, energy, effort and financial resources.

Better Tips: This tip will progress you further into implementing the lesson idea. More time and cost may be involved in this step.

Best Tips: When you are ready, this tip will give you ideas to help implement the lesson ideas in a more extensive fashion. This could mean significant investment of time, energy, effort, and financial resources.

LESSON 2:

"Every cell in your body is eavesdropping on your thoughts!" - Dr. Patrick Quillin

Did you know that your body responds to the way you think, feel or imagine?

Good: When you have a negative thought, immediately stop it in its tracks and say out loud "That thought has no hold on me." Make an index card with notes on how you will be healed and whole. Include a scripture reference to read. Read every day.

Better: Start a gratitude journal that you will begin everyday with. Write "Today, I am grateful for...." and journal about the things you are most grateful for. Choose life.

Best: Read one of the books recommended in the lesson to further your belief that you can heal.
- Brenda Stockdale's book, *You Can Beat the Odds*
- Dr. Caroline Leaf's book, *Switch On Your Brain: The Key to Peak Happiness, Thinking, and Health*
- Mark Rutland's book, *Courage to Be Healed: Finding Hope to Restore Your Soul*

DISCUSSION QUESTIONS/ACTION STEPS:

1. Write three attitudes or beliefs you foresee hampering your healing and share with someone sitting near you. For example: My family and I love unhealthy fried foods. I don't know enough. There isn't another doctor to help me.

   REFRAME: How can you reframe those three beliefs/thoughts that are hampering your healing? For example: Instead of saying: "My family and I love unhealthy fried foods." Your reframed thought might be "I can't wait to try new foods that will help heal my body".

   _____
   _____
   _____

2. How will you begin to shift your thoughts? For example: I will pay more attention to my thoughts and words seeking to focus on things that are helpful and not hurtful.

   _____
   _____
   _____

3. What is your goal for this month? What are some obstacles? Tell someone in the group what you want to accomplish and how you plan to do it.

   _____
   _____
   _____

4. Who are some of your favorite local doctors who use or are open to more natural healing approaches and techniques?

   _____
   _____
   _____

CONNECT:

As a participant in a HealingStrong™ group, you have much to take advantage of in your healing journey. Our meetings are just a part of helping you on a consistent basis. Review these resources for things that can help Rebuild, Renew, and Refresh you all month long!

HealingStrong™ website: http://healingstrong.org
HealingStrong™ Facebook page: http://www.facebook.com/healingstrong/
HealingStrong™ Instagram page: https://www.instagram.com/healingstrongofficial/
HealingStrong™ I AM HealingStrong™ Podcast page: https://healingstrong.org/podcast
HealingStrong™ Start Here: https://healingstrong.org/start-here

Remember: "Fear is detrimental to healing, but affirmations based on God's Word help us replace it with courage and strength."

FIYAA AFFIRMATIONS

I will:

- **Forgive** myself and others.
- **Invite** God into all aspects of my life and healing.
- **Yield** to the needs of my body during this healing season.
- **Accept** my diagnosis and symptoms as temporary.
- **Abandon** negative expectations and think possibilities.

WWW.HEALINGSTRONG.ORG

Being a faith-based organization, we are not only passionate about your present healing journey, but also passionate about your eternal destiny as well. Of course, there will come an end to this life for all of us. We want to make sure that we have shared with you how to know that your eternal destiny is in heaven with our Creator, the One who formed you, loves you, and made a simple way for you to know for certain. If you are not a believer in Jesus Christ and would like to learn more about His saving grace, please see these resources: https://healingstrong.org/refresh

NOTES

Lesson 2 Additional Resources for Further Use

None at this time

I find true happiness when I walk in the light of God's true presence.

Read: Psalm: 16:11

healingstrong

Raw Brussel Sprout Salad
by Sandra Campbell

- 1 package Brussel sprouts, cored and sliced very thin
- 1 Tablespoon Hemp Seeds
- 1 small handful raw cashews, chopped
- 2 Tablespoons raw pumpkin seeds
- 1 lemon, juiced
- ¼ cup extra virgin olive oil

Make a dressing of the lemon juice and olive oil, set aside. Combine all other ingredients in a bowl and toss well to combine. Add a little of the dressing at a time to taste. Season with Himalayan Sea Salt.

Good source of Vitamins A, C, K and B6. Contains riboflavin, iron, magnesium, thiamin, folate, potassium, manganese, and copper. Excellent source of protein. Hemp contains all the essential amino and fatty acids necessary to maintain healthy human life.

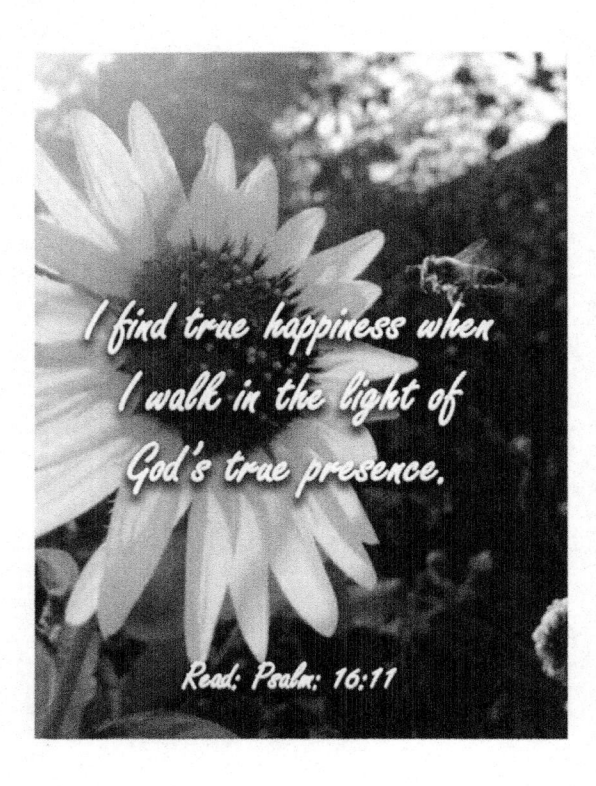

Dear Heavenly Father,

I ask You to bring grace and comfort to me and my family. Life is not perfect or smooth. Trials come, but we are comforted knowing that You are with us. Yes, I believe in Your plan of good! Storms come not to harm us, but to cause a deeper faith in You. Show us, oh, God the ways of Your plan. We love and believe in You! Grow us in our faith – so deep – so strong – that it is all we need.

Comfort Blessing by Kirsti A. Dyer, M.D.

May you see the light in the darkness during these challenging times.

May you feel the loving presence of those who hold you in their thoughts and prayers.

May your spirit find what it needs to sustain you on this journey.

May you discover your inner strength and face all difficulties with dignity and grace.

May you be filled with comfort, love, strength, grace, and a lasting sense of peace.

Thank you for the promises in Your Word. Amen.

Lesson 3:
Cancer Basics and First Steps Towards Healing

> **NOTE:** The full Participant Guide is available for download at our Start Here Page https://healingstrong.org/start-here. Please also review our full disclaimer for HealingStrong™ at: https://healingstrong.org/start-here.

LESSON OBJECTIVES & KEY CONCEPTS

Take Away/Objective:

What is cancer and what causes cancer? How does your immune system handle it? What impact does changing to a plant-based diet have on cancer and your body?

Key Concepts:

- Cancer develops when the body begins to group large amounts of mutated cells into tumors that can spread and begin to cause problems to healthy body function.

- Cancer is your body sending a message that you are not giving it what it needs to thrive OR giving it too much of what is harmful (this can be spiritual, nutritional, emotional, etc.).

- Eating a diet full of meat, processed and fried foods, sugar, artificial sweeteners, food dyes, fast food, and caffeine negatively affects the body. Many of these effects gradually lead to chronic illnesses and cancer.

- A diet high in raw, organic vegetables and fruits has cleansing, anti-cancer, anti-inflammatory, healing effects on the body.

DISCUSSION POINTS

***Note to the Reader: Although lessons are geared towards healing from cancer, these lessons are educational in nature and offer information that will equip and empower you with health choices and action steps that you can take that may benefit your overall well-being. If you are on a healing protocol, whether preventative in nature, or treatment that is conventional, holistic or integrative, the principles taught in these lessons may be applied towards a supportive plan for many health challenges.

Introduction: Some of us are here today because we are dealing with a surprise cancer diagnosis. Some of us might be dealing with other chronic illnesses that conventional medicine hasn't helped much, or you desire to prevent such illnesses. Today we're going to take a closer look at what causes chronic disease and talk about some basic changes we can make now. Although we focus on cancer, please know that all chronic disease can be helped with these healing strategies. By starting at cancer and working backwards, we hope to help reveal habits that lead to poor health, encouraging prevention for our future. As in Lesson 2 (Building Confidence: Your Right to Take Charge of Your Health), your BELIEF about healing can make or break your healing results. LEARNING this information about cancer and disease formation can help you see that it is not random. Also, you can learn how to support and empower your body to reverse this situation.

What Causes Chronic Disease and Cancer?
- Plenty of experts agree, we don't just get cancer randomly or from bad luck.
- Cancer is CAUSED through our day-to-day choices. Watch Chris Beat Cancer's first video for free for understanding this concept. https://healingstrong.org/resources
- According to the American Association of Pharmaceutical Scientists:
"Cancer is a preventable disease that requires major lifestyle changes. Only 5-10% of all cancer cases can be attributed to genetic defects, whereas the remaining 90-95% have their roots in the environment and lifestyle". https://pubmed.ncbi.nlm.nih.gov/-18626751/

Cancer and The Immune System
- To deactivate the stigma of cancer being a *death sentence*, it is very important to learn what it is, what causes it, and how the immune system handles it.
- Daily unhealthy choices can trigger our normal cells into mutating, primarily due to damaged DNA within them. These mutated cancer cells do not know when to quit and continue multiplying without dying. A healthy immune system combats these out-of-control cells, but if it is chronically weakened, these cell numbers can get out of control.

- At some point, these cancer cells become so numerous they become a mass that you may feel, or is detected on a mammogram or CT scan. This is what we know as a TUMOR, and it is at this point that cancer is usually diagnosed.
- As the tumor grows, it needs additional energy sources, primarily SUGAR, and begins to grow its own new blood vessels in search of energy supply in a process called ANGIOGENESIS. This is how cancer spreads to other parts of the body as it travels through your bloodstream through these newly formed blood vessels. In most cases, this process takes YEARS to happen.
- Here is an article on the impact of sugar on cancer cells. https://www.konstantinic-center.org/en/cancer-cells-are-fed-by-sugar-says-john-hopkins-research/
- Here is a video on how to eat to starve cancer by Dr. Li. https://www.youtube.com/watch?v=B9bDZ5-zPtY&t=5s
- It is fair to say that anyone with cancer or other disease has a weakened immune system caused by a combination of many factors: our poor diets, lack of sleep, toxic use of chemicals, negative thinking, stress, and/or overuse of pharmaceuticals and other harmful substances.

Changing Your Diet
- The very first, and sometimes hardest, lifestyle change is your diet.
- The condition of our bodies is dependent on the quality of the foods we eat, as well as our toxic exposure.
- No matter what treatment plan you choose, changing your lifestyle towards a diet rich in plant-based, organic, whole foods is a MUST.
- Focusing for a season on micro-nutrient dense foods (fruits and vegetables) and reducing or eliminating meats for a season will give your digestion a break and also promote healing.
- It is important to note that there are varying schools of thought regarding the choice to go completely vegan (no meat, fish, dairy, etc.) or allow clean meats such as fish in a healing diet. The authors of this resource believe there is a season of eliminating meats and supporting the body with nutrient rich clean foods, promoting easier digestion and detoxification. That season may vary depending on the individual and his/her needs.
- According to Dr. Joel Furhman's Eat to Live, some of the most beneficial foods for healing and preventing cancer are green vegetables, beans, onions, berries and seeds.
- Dr. Furhman's Aggregate Nutrient Density Index (ANDI) scoring system rates foods according to the concentration of micronutrients per calorie. (https://www.drfuhrman.com/learn/library/articles/95/_andi-food-scores-rating-the-nutrient-density-of-foodslibrary/)

- God gave us a clue when he created people. He placed them in a GARDEN. He told them what to eat, and it could all be grown right where they were. He even put it in the very first chapter of his Word so we couldn't miss it!

"Then God said, 'I give you every seed-bearing plant on the face of the whole earth and every tree that has fruit with seed in it. They will be yours for food.'" Genesis 1:29 (NIV)

- There are other verses in the Scriptures, providing insight on the original plan for food, as well as various herbs listed for healing. (https://www.openbible.info/topics/-herbs_for_healing)
- How is it possible so many overlook this? Our culture has a pretty strong pull on us, and we are several generations into a lifestyle of supermarket dependence. This dependence has us focused on recipes made from processed food, and we often don't even know what to do with fresh produce.
- For the body to heal, we have to stay away from processed foods. The fewer the ingredients, the better.
- Anything with a long shelf-life, due to processed additives, is a food to avoid
- Many of us grew up eating canned soups, boxed pastas, instant side dishes, and microwave dinners. Our meat came from factory farms where animals live and die within a 3-foot radius and are pumped with antibiotics and growth hormones.
- RELEARN and RETRAIN our belief system about food.
- It is not just for enjoyment and to keep us alive.
- Food is actual medicine to help the body thrive, not simply survive with illness.
- Hippocrates, who is considered the father of modern medicine, stated:

"Let food be thy medicine and medicine be thy food." He also said, "Keep away from the chemist's pot if you can heal from food."

- Today's doctors still take the Hippocratic Oath. What Hippocrates taught still stands true today, but most run to the chemist pot (pharmaceuticals) without first examining what we are putting in and on our body.
- It has been said by an unknown source, "What you choose to put in your body is either feeding it, OR it is feeding your disease" (cancer, heart disease, diabetes, etc.).
- A great program to review for how to eat is Chris Wark's SquareOne program. You can find the materials at this link for purchase for a small fee. He also has twice a year free viewing of the program available. https://healingstrong.org/resources

Eat an Abundance of These Foods to Promote Healing
A therapeutic healing diet will have these components:
- Cleanses the body and intestines
- Detoxifies the liver and major organs
- Promotes anti-angiogenesis
- Promotes apoptosis, which is defined as cancer cell die-off
- Nourishes cells, tissues, and organs to heal the body and give energy
- Low or completely clear of sugar, processed foods, meat, caffeine, and wheat products

If you are healing from cancer or other disease, focus on getting 100% (or as close as possible) of raw and organic plants, as well as mostly non-starchy vegetables into your body. This can be in the form of juicing, smoothies, and salads. Cortney Campbell, The Anti-Cancer Mom, talks about many of these items in her post - http://www.anticancermom.com/organic-raw-vegan-diet. You can track the foods and supplements you take by using the food and action supplement chart. Your group leader can provide you a copy.

Organic Food
- When reclaiming your health with food as your medicine, you want your food to be as pure as possible
- Buying organic is important to the anti-cancer diet or any healthy lifestyle and ensures that you are not getting a genetically modified (GMO) product. It is common knowledge that when pesticides are sprayed on produce, many of those fruits and vegetables actually absorb the chemicals. They essentially become a part of the fruit or vegetable. When reclaiming your health with food as your medicine, you want your food to be as pure as possible.
- When pesticides are sprayed on produce, many of those fruits and vegetables actually absorb the chemicals.
- EWG's Dirty Dozen™, chemical prone fruits and veggies: peaches, apples, bell peppers, celery, nectarines, strawberries. cherries, pears, grapes, spinach, kale/greens, and tomatoes. Some studies also include blueberries. https://www.ewg.org/food-news/dirty-dozen.php
- If buying organic is difficult due to cost or availability, focus on "good, better, best". Start with what you can like replacing the items on the dirty dozen list with organic first.

Raw Food
- When we cook food, we destroy a lot of its natural enzymes.
- Enzymes are naturally occurring in raw fruits and vegetables and help us to digest them much easier, rather than forcing the digestive system to do all the work.
- Plant products practically digest themselves and contain fiber to clean out your colon, aiding in detoxification and allowing for maximum absorption of nutrients.
- Living, raw foods also contain the optimal amount of vitamins and minerals in forms readily used by the body.
- Uncooked fruits and veggies boost your body's alkalinity, which has been shown to deter cancer and other diseases that thrive in an acidic environment.

- There are some people who have digestive difficulties and might find a plant-based diet rich in raw foods challenging at first. Healing a sick gut is important and may require easing into a raw diet by first addressing the gut.
- For more information about healing a sick gut, we recommend you read: *GAPS Diet (Gut and Psychology Syndrome by Dr. Natasha Campbell-McBride, MD).*

Gut Healing Food/Fermented Food
- Focusing on having healthy gut flora or bacteria is important when on a healing protocol.
- Take a daily probiotic (see Lesson 4, Helpful Supplements and What Not To Eat When Healing).
- Eat fermented food and drinks daily examples: sauerkraut, veggie kraut, kombucha, miso, and others.

Superfood
- Garlic, berries, onions, dark leafy greens, cruciferous vegetables such as cabbage, broccoli, brussels sprouts, and cauliflower, turmeric, and carrots are considered superfoods due to their disease fighting properties.
- Spirulina, acai, mangosteen, maca powder, raw cacao, and goji berries are also full of nutrients.

Anti-Angiogenesis Food
- These foods have discouraging effects on the formation of new blood vessels.
- By stopping this process, we starve the tumor of its energy to grow and spread.
- Eat an abundance of these foods, including all berries, green tea, maitake mushrooms, shiitake mushrooms, chaga mushrooms, turmeric, red grapes, pineapple, kale, garlic, dark leafy greens, onions, and broccoli sprouts. https://blog.ted.com/dr_william_lis/
- Cinnamon extract also suppresses tumor progression by inhibiting angiogenesis, or new blood vessels from forming around the cancer. https://www.ncbi.nlm.nih.gov/pmc/articles/PMC2920880/

Smoothies
- These can be a time saver and easy on the go meal.
- They will help you get enough calories to maintain your weight while eating a mostly plant-based diet.
- Smoothies also fill your belly and digest slowly, allowing a longer feeling of fullness.
- Vegetables blend well in a smoothie with an apple or a banana to help enliven the flavor.
- You can add a natural, organic, vegan protein with just one scoop of powder.
- You can also use healthy oils and fats, such as: coconut oil, flaxseed oil, nuts, and avocado.
- Store smoothies in a 32 oz canning mason jar or BPA-free Nalgene brand bottle.
- A great site to find ideas and recipes is https://simplegreensmoothies.com. You can also search for "plant based smoothies" and find lots of great options for your taste.

Juicing

- Juicing is a large part of many natural cancer treatments including the Gerson Protocol (see Lesson 5, 7 Steps for Choosing a Non-Toxic Protocol).
- Eating solid food requires many hours of digestion before the nutrients are available to our tissues and cells. Removing fiber enables the juices to be assimilated quickly into the body.
- By juicing vegetables and removing the fiber, your intestines are able to digest and soak in ALL the vitamins and minerals directly into the bloodstream without having to work through the fiber.
- Drinking up to eight 8 ounce juices a day is common while healing naturally.
- Many vegetables can be juiced, but especially popular when healing are carrots, celery, beets, ginger, kale, chard, spinach, cabbage, broccoli, and green apples.
- The Juice Lady, Cherie Calbom examines juicing and various juice combinations at https://www.juiceladycherie.com/Juice/recipes/.
- Cherie and Fr. John Calbom offer an intensive five day juice and raw retreat to jumpstart healing. For more information: https://juiceladycherie.com/juice-health-retreats/
- See also, one of our favorite documentaries, *Fat, Sick and Nearly Dead.* https://www.rebootwithjoe.com/joes-films/
- Chris has an article and the details on his juice recipe at this link. https://www.chrisbeatcancer.com/i-juiced-to-beat-cancer-and-turned-orange/
- Watch a video of Suzy talking with Cherie about Juicing tips on our Refresh tab at the bottom of the page. https://healingstrong.org/rebuild
- Other videos on juicing are available on the **HealingStrong™** website:. Look at the Healing Journey Jumpstart video on Juicing your Way to Health. https://healing-strong.org/start-here

Salads

- Salads can be delicious when on an anti-cancer diet.
- Make a large nutrient dense salad daily.
- Helps ensure you will be ingesting micro-nutrients that are disease fighting.
- Chopping a salad of dark green, leafy, vegetables and adding apple cider vinegar, flax oil, and nutritional yeast can jazz it up.
- Add protein with nuts, seeds, avocado, carrots, broccoli, kale, cabbage, onions, beans, or a bit of almond butter.
- Seeds help facilitate phyto-chemical absorption.
- A delicious salad recipe can be found at: http://www.chrisbeatcancer.com/the-giant-cancer-fighting-salad
- Here is an option for making a salad in a jar. https://plantbasedscotty.com/5-healthy-mason-jar-salad-recipes-for-the-week

Good, Better, Best Tips

Introduction for section on Good Better Best:

As each lesson concludes, we want to leave you with an idea(s) for how to implement a suggestion from the lesson in an incremental fashion that meets your needs and abilities. Each lesson will give you ideas that are "Good, Better, and Best".

Good Tips: A perfect way to get started implementing healthier healing options. This tip will be less involved from both a time, energy, effort and financial resources.

Better Tips: This tip will progress you further into implementing the lesson idea. More time and cost may be involved in this step.

Best Tips: When you are ready, this tip will give you ideas to help implement the lesson ideas in a more extensive fashion. This could mean significant investment of time, energy, effort, and financial resources.

LESSON 3:

A diet rich in plant-based whole foods can provide you with the proper nutrients necessary when you are focused on a healing protocol.

Good: Start implementing a plant-based diet by focusing on breakfast first. Find a new breakfast choice and implement it! Oatmeal is a great option. https://www.chrisbeatcancer.com/how-to-supercharge-your-oatmeal/

Better: Add fresh fruits and vegetables into your diet daily through routines such as cut up strawberries or fresh blueberries added to your oatmeal each morning.

Best: To turbo charge your nutrient intake each day, add fresh juices that you make with organic vegetables and fruits. (Example of juice recipe: 3 organic carrots, one green apple, ½ lemon, 1 swiss chard leaf, 1 thumb-size of ginger)

DISCUSSION QUESTIONS/ACTION STEPS

1. How does everyone feel about seeing cancer as a symptom of a lifestyle problem rather than a disease we have little control over?

   _____
   _____
   _____

2. On a scale of 1-10 with 1 being the worst, how would you rate your current diet? Why?

   _____
   _____
   _____

3. What is one doable step you could take today to improve your diet? Who could help encourage you?

   _____
   _____
   _____

4. What do you foresee being the biggest roadblock to improving your diet? Discuss strategies to overcome this.

   _____
   _____
   _____

5. What are your favorite health food stores in the area?

   _____
   _____
   _____

CONNECT:

As a participant in a HealingStrong™ group, you have much to take advantage of in your healing journey. Our meetings are just a part of helping you on a consistent basis. Review these resources for things that can help Rebuild, Renew, and Refresh you all month long!

HealingStrong™ website: http://healingstrong.org
HealingStrong™ Facebook page: http://www.facebook.com/healingstrong/
HealingStrong™ Instagram page: https://www.instagram.com/healingstrongofficial/
HealingStrong™ I AM HealingStrong™ Podcast page: https://healingstrong.org/podcast
HealingStrong™ Start Here: https://healingstrong.org/start-here

Remember: "Fear is detrimental to healing, but affirmations based on God's Word help us replace it with courage and strength."

FIYAA AFFIRMATIONS

I will:

- **Forgive** myself and others.
- **Invite** God into all aspects of my life and healing.
- **Yield** to the needs of my body during this healing season.
- **Accept** my diagnosis and symptoms as temporary
- **Abandon** negative expectations and think possibilities.

WWW.HEALINGSTRONG.ORG

Being a faith-based organization, we are not only passionate about your present healing journey, but also passionate about your eternal destiny as well. Of course, there will come an end to this life for all of us. We want to make sure that we have shared with you how to know that your eternal destiny is in heaven with our Creator, the One who formed you, loves you, and made a simple way for you to know for certain. If you are not a believer in Jesus Christ and would like to learn more about His saving grace, please see these resources: https://healingstrong.org/refresh

NOTES

Lesson 3 Additional Resources for Further Use

"Breakthrough Study Shows Personalised Nutrition Future for Probiotics." *NutraIngredients.com*. 16 Dec. 2015. Web. <https://www.nutraingredients.com/Article/2010/09/15/Breakthrough-study-shows-personalised-nutrition-future-for-probiotics#>

Campbell, T. Colin, and Thomas M. Campbell. ***The China Study: The Most Comprehensive Study of Nutrition Ever Conducted and the Startling Implications for Diet, Weight Loss and Long-term Health***. Dallas, Tex.: BenBella, 2005. Print.

"DETOX - Health Starts With Your Diet - Green Drink Diaries." *Green Drink Diaries*. 1 Feb. 2011. Web. <http://www.anticancermom.com/detox-health-starts-with-your-diet/.>

Desaulniers, Veronique. ***Heal Breast Cancer Naturally: 7 Essential Steps to Beating Breast Cancer***. *Dr. Veronique Desaulniers*. 2019. Print.

"Dietary Supplements, Nutraceuticals, Functional Foods, Health Ingredients, Herbals."

NutraIngredients.com. 16 Dec. 2015. Web. <http://www.nutraingredients.com/.>

"Dr. Joel Fuhrman: 3 Foods You Should Eat Every Day." *YouTube*. YouTube. 16 Dec. 2015. Web. <https:// https://www.youtube.com/watch?v=WSUfgej-CF0.>

"Dr. Stephen Sinatra's Informational Site - Heart MD Institute." *Dr. Stephen Sinatra's Informational Site - Heart MD Institute*. 16 Dec. 2015. Web. <https://heartmdinstitute.com/.>

"Eat to Beat Disease." *Eat to Beat: Home*. 16 Dec. 2015. Web. <http://www.eattobeat.org.>

"Everything You HAVE TO KNOW about Dangerous Genetically Modified Foods." *Vimeo*. 16 Dec. 2015. Web. <https://vimeo.com/6575475.>

Fuhrman, Joel. ***Eat to Live: The Amazing Nutrient-rich Program for Fast and Sustained Weight Loss***. Rev. ed. New York: Little, Brown, 2011. Print.

Forks Over Knives. Dir. Lee Fulkerson. Monica Beach Media, 2011.

<https://www.forksoverknives.com/the-film/>

<https://www.forksoverknives.com>

Gerson, Charlotte, and Beata Bishop. *Healing the Gerson Way: Defeating Cancer and Other Chronic Diseases*. New ed. Carmel, CA: Gerson Health Media, 2010. Print.

"My Food DETOX and CHECK THAT LABEL! - Green Drink Diaries." *Green Drink Diaries.* 2 Feb. 2011. 16 Dec. 2015. Web. <http://www.anticancermom.com/my-food-detox-and-check-that-label/>

"Sample One Day Menu for a Gerson Therapy Patient." 16 Dec. 2015. Web. <https://gerson.org/wp-content/uploads/2020/02/Gerson-Cookbook-Sample-Menu-and-Shopping-List.pdf>

Walker, N. W. *Fresh Vegetable and Fruit Juices: What's Missing in Your Body?* Rev. ed. Phoenix, Ariz.: [Norwalk], 1978. Print.

> **God is with me in times of trouble.**
> Read: Psalm 46:1

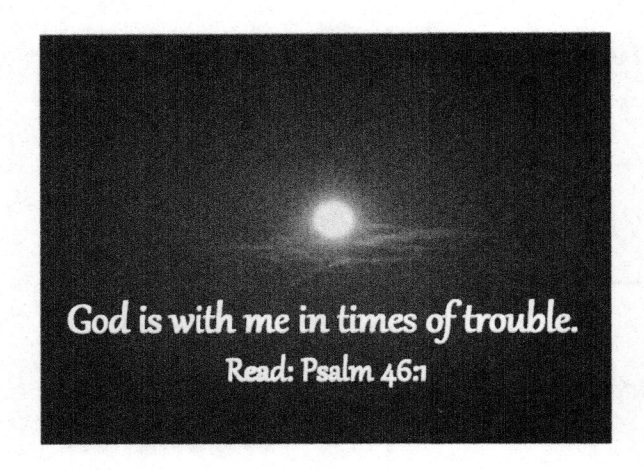

Dear Heavenly Father,

I pray reminders from YOU in Your Word that:

- **YOUR compassion and love never fail.** Lamentations 3:22
- **YOU created me in YOUR image.** Genesis 1:27
- **YOU count me precious and honored in Your sight, and You love me.** Isaiah 43:4
- **YOUR protection covers me from my enemies.** Psalm 59:1

Please, Lord, help me to know Your truths in Your Word that I will hear Your voice and follow the pathway that You have set for me. For You say, *"When a man's ways please the Lord, He makes even His enemies to be at peace with Him."* Proverbs 16:7

In Jesus' name I pray. Amen.

Quinoa Salad
by Sandra Campbell

- 4 cups water
- 2 cups quinoa, dry
- 1 cucumber, diced
- 1 tomato, diced
- 1 handful parsley, chopped
- 1 green onion, sliced thin, tops included
- 1 lemon, juiced
- ½ cup extra virgin olive oil
- ¼ cup red wine vinegar

Cook quinoa in boiling water according to package directions. While quinoa is cooking, whisk together lemon juice, olive oil and vinegar. Set aside. When quinoa is done, put it in a large bowl and add all other ingredients. Toss with dressing and season with salt and pepper to taste.

Good source of Vitamins E, B6, A, C and K. Contains calcium, iron, riboflavin, manganese, phosphorus, magnesium, copper, zinc and folate. Supplies dietary fiber. Quinoa is a high quality protein.

Lesson 4:
Helpful Supplements and What Not to Eat When Healing

> **NOTE:** The full Participant Guide is available for download at our Start Here Page https://healingstrong.org/start-here. Please also review our full disclaimer for Healing-Strong™ at: https://healingstrong.org/start-here.

LESSON OBJECTIVES & KEY CONCEPTS

Take Away/Objective:

Understand common dietary deficiencies that people with chronic disease tend to have. Understand how we should use supplements when we are healing. Learn about the most common foods that impede nutrient absorption.

Key Concepts:

- Supplements help you achieve optimum health by bridging the gap of any functional deficiencies.

- Supplements can be costly and being a well-informed self-advocate will help you to determine where you should place your focus.

- Eating a healthy diet rich in vitamins and nutrients obtained from organic, whole foods should be your primary source; however, optimum health for an individual suffering from disease means supplementing where deficient.

- It is important to understand how to recognize good quality supplements.

- Avoiding foods that impede nutrient absorption and healing is important on your healing journey.

DISCUSSION POINTS

***Note to the Reader: Although lessons are geared towards healing from cancer, these lessons are educational in nature and offer information that will equip and empower you with health choices and action steps that you can take that may benefit your overall well-being. If you are on a healing protocol, whether preventative in nature, or treatment that is conventional, holistic or integrative, the principles taught in these lessons may be applied towards a supportive plan for many health challenges.

Introduction: Today, we are going to talk about how you can enhance your healing diet with the most popular and notable nutritional supplements, as well as talk about foods and additives to avoid, especially in a healing season. There are thousands of supplements which could be beneficial when healing, but determining the best ones for you can be frustrating. Oftentimes, people begin taking supplements because someone recommended it, an advertisement online or the television prompted you to buy it, or maybe you were told it was mission critical for you to take the supplement without full knowledge of why. Before you know it, you have a bin of half empty supplement containers!

Common Dietary Deficiencies

It is important in your decision to add supplements to your diet to understand that the natural form of nutrition is always best. Ensure that you are adding whole food plant based nutrition to your diet (i.e.: eating fruits and vegetables everyday).

Also, blood tests can help determine if you are truly deficient in some key areas like Vitamin D, B, and many others. Talk with your healthcare provider about having testing done to understand your deficiencies and to ensure you are taking the correct dosage. Make sure that you start with adding nutrients in plant-based food form first! Drinking your Vitamin C and using sunshine for your Vitamin D are important. Check out this article and graphic to understand how to get your vitamins from our plant based food sources. https://guidetovegan.com/vegan-nutrition/ See this article to understand some deficiencies. https://www.nature.com/articles/nrc886

Supplements

How do you choose the optimal supplement for you?

Research those supplements that will support your unique case (while working with a knowledgeable practitioner). Deane Alban with Be Brain Fit has written an article that has good direction on choosing supplements. We have listed some of those and other sources of information as you start your journey on choosing supplements below. See: https://bebrainfit.com/choose-nutritional-supplements/

Chris Wark also has a great video on the supplements that he uses.

- https://www.chrisbeatcancer.com/supplements-for-super-immunity/
- https://www.chrisbeatcancer.com/category/products/supplements/

Kris Carr, stage 4 cancer thriver and author of Crazy Sexy Cancer Tips, also discusses supplements in this article:

- https://kriscarr.com/blog/cancer-supplements/

Healthline Article:

- https://www.healthline.com/health/anti-cancer-supplements

Here are some things to consider when purchasing supplements:

1. Nutrient Form - Read labels carefully to see what nutrient forms are included. These are listed in parentheses after the name of the nutrient. Natural forms of the nutrients are usually easier for the body to use than synthetic forms.
2. Dosage Level - Does the supplement have an adequate amount of the nutrient to actually improve your health?
3. Quality - Good companies use independent research to verify quality, formulation, and effectiveness. They ensure their ingredients are free of contaminants and have excellent quality-control measures. It is important to do your own research into the companies from which you are considering purchasing.
4. Price - Cheap prices usually mean cheap ingredients; however, there are expensive products that also can be ineffective. Consumerlab.com specializes in testing products for quality and potency.
5. Expiration Dates - Look for products that offer this date. The FDA doesn't require it, but most reputable companies will provide it for you.
6. Label Red Flags and Other Ingredients - Look for "red flags" on labels —sugar, artificial coloring and flavoring, preservatives, and additives such as shellac, chlorine, and other chemicals should be avoided.

Recommendations for Supplements for Immune system support:
please discuss your individualized dosage with your practitioner

1. Iodine - (There are risks to taking too much iodine, so this should be researched, monitored by requesting an iodine loading kit, and discussed with your practitioner). Iodine deficiency has become a worldwide epidemic. Iodine is an important nutrient that can support brain development and ensure proper thyroid function (which keeps cells healthy). We recommend the following resource for further reading: The Iodine Crisis by Lynne Farrow http://lynnefarrow.net/book.html
2. CoEnzyme Q-10 - acts as an antioxidant
3. Pancreatin (Pancreatic Enzymes) - aids in digestion - See Lesson 6 (Healing Protocols and Adjunct Therapies) or https://thegonzalezprotocol.com/videos/pancreatic-enzymes-as-cancer-treatment/

4. Probiotic capsules: According to Nutraingredients.com, consumption of a dairy drink containing three strains of probiotic bacteria was associated with changes in the activity of hundreds of genes, with the changes resembling the effects of certain medicines in the human body, including medicines that positively influence the immune system and those for lowering blood pressure. https://www.nutraingredients.com/Article/2010/09/15/Breakthrough-study-shows-personalised-nutrition-future-for-probiotics
5. Digestive Enzymes - aids in digestion
6. Selenium - protects against cell damage - https://draxe.com/nutrition/selenium-benefits/
7. Beta-1, 3D Glucan - See this great article on Beta-1 glucan. Helps the immune system fight cancer cells. http://www.anticancermom.com/beta-1-3-d-glucan/
8. Vitamin D3 - promote cancer cell death and decrease growth of cancer cells
9. Curcumin/Turmeric - reduces inflammation
10. Super green powder supplement (organic, if possible) - reduces inflammation
11. Vitamin C - kills cancer cells
12. Magnesium - improves the ability of the immune system to eliminate infected and cancerous cells
13. Astragalus - may help shrink tumors

Tips for Managing Supplements:

Taking a large number of supplements can be overwhelming. Using a pill organizer and/or a pill reminder app is a great way to manage a complex regimen.

- You can find samples of pill organizers on Amazon. https://www.amazon.com/gp/product/B082BFKNTR/ref=ppx_yo_dt_b_search_asin_title?ie=UTF8&psc=1
- Here is an example of a pill reminder. Many of the apps are free. https://www.aidaorganizer.com/mac/pillsreminder.html
- It could be beneficial to rotate supplements. This could include changing brands, rotating types you are taking, etc. It would be important to discuss this with your doctor. https://www.theforkclinic.com/post/avoiding-supplement-overload

What Not to Eat When Healing

Dr. Axe notes, "Cancer is a systemic disease with various causes, some of which include a poor diet, toxin exposure, nutrient deficiencies and to some extent genetics. One extremely important way to prevent and/or treat cancer is nutritionally, through eating a nutrient-dense diet full of cancer-fighting foods and avoiding things that are known to increase cancer risk."

He also notes, "Inflammation is the underlying issue that dictates cancerous tumor initiation, progression and growth. Studies suggest that 30 percent to 40 percent of all kinds of cancer can be prevented with a healthy lifestyle and dietary measures! And other sources claim that this number is in fact much higher, with around 75 percent of cancer cases being lifestyle-related." See: https://draxe.com/nutrition/cancer-fighting-foods/

Suggestions for how to start adjusting your diet:
- Eliminate packaged foods in cans, bags, boxes, and bottles.
- Cut out meat and dairy as many healing protocols for cancer suggest this.**
- If you choose to continue to eat dairy or meat, we highly recommend finding a non-pasteurized, raw milk from a local, organic farmer, and choosing organic, pasture raised meats.**
- All pork should be avoided.
- Taking high doses of digestive enzymes is very important to aid in digestion.
- In order to maximize the plant-based nutrients, consider juicing, smoothies and an abundance of green salads and vegetables.

**HealingStrong™ believes cutting out meat (at least for a season) is important due to the energy it takes your body to digest and process animal based proteins. Focusing on improved absorption of the nutrients offered in plant-based foods is our recommendation for a season and that season may last months, or years. This doesn't mean you have to become a vegan forever, but we do encourage you to prayerfully consider getting your protein and nutrients from plants. If you choose to eat meat, fish is the easiest meat to digest, then chicken, then beef.

Foods to Eliminate or Limit

We ask that you do your own research about these items in healing diets and pray through your decision. Many recognized healing protocols for cancer suggest at least a season of eliminating the items below from your diet:

Isolated refined white sugar

- Sugar is one of the most addictive substances in the world. It has serious effects on your brain function and your psyche.
- Sugar promotes cancer growth, spikes your insulin, contributes to inflammation, damages skin collagen, promotes wrinkles, increases appetite, depletes the body of B vitamins, and causes joint degeneration.
- The 1931 Nobel laureate in medicine, German Otto Warburg, Ph.D., first discovered that cancer cells metabolize differently than healthy cells. He discovered that glucose fuels cancer cells, compared to normal tissues fueled by oxygen. See: http://www.cancertutor.com/hydrazine/ (Sugar fuels cancer, as do carbohydrates, alcohol, and other types of sugar. This statement may create controversy among many. We encourage you to read and research why sugar fuels cancer and should be eliminated as much as possible.)
- All grains, including bread, pasta, alcohol, and high sugar fruits turn into glucose in the blood when metabolized, and should be avoided during a healing season.
- To go from "good" to "better", consider using maple syrup or eating a date where you might have used sugar in the past. Best case scenario is to cut out your sugar completely, especially during a healing season.
- HealingStrong™ founder, Suzy Griswold, has a book that talks about the AHA moments of her cancer journey. This includes the AHA Moment on Sugar feeds cancer. See: https://healingstrong.org/resources

- See these articles for the different types of ways sugar is listed on food labels.
  https://healthyeating.sfgate.com/different-words-sugar-food-labels-8373.html
  https://www.virtahealth.com/blog/names-for-sugar

Meat and Dairy

- Digesting animal products requires your body to work harder. If your body is striving to heal cancer, you need all the energy and enzymes you have to do just that.
- Plant products practically digest themselves and contain tons of fiber to clean out your colon to allow for optimal absorption of nutrients.
- Most dairy products are also "dead" of their enzymes since many of their nutrients have been destroyed in the pasteurization process.
- If you are dealing with chronic illness, and especially cancer, you need to stay clear of all animal products, at least for a season of initial healing, then you can work with your doctor as to what and how much to add back into your diet (especially if weight loss is an issue).

High Fructose Corn Syrup (HFCS)

- HFCS is toxic to the liver, increases inflammation, bodily stress, weight gain, and causes sudden insulin surges, which over time, can lead to type 2 diabetes.

Hydrogenated/Partially Hydrogenated Oils (Trans Fats)

- Your body doesn't know what to do with trans fat, since it is altered in a lab by adding additional hydrogen to a fat molecule. This results in solid fat with a longer shelf life, which appeals to frugal companies.
- Although trans fats are now outlawed, they may still appear in some foods. See:
  https://www.healthline.com/nutrition/trans-fat-foods#basics

MSG

- Monosodium glutamate (MSG) is a chemical that has been associated with reproductive disorders, migraine headaches and decreased fertility. MSG is used in many foods as a taste enhancer.
- MSG can also be referred to as yeast extract, hydrolyzed protein, and soy protein isolate. See a detailed list here: https://www.hungryforchange.tv/article/sneaky-names-for-msg-check-your-labels

Sodium Nitrate

- Sodium Nitrate is a preservative, coloring and flavoring commonly added to bacon, ham, hot dogs, lunch meats, and smoked fish.
- Studies have linked eating it to various types of cancer. One way to avoid nitrites is to avoid eating processed pork products, which have very little nutritional benefits compared to the risks.

Processed Soy
- Stick to fermented organic soy products or seitan and avoid all others, avoid processed soy, and soy "fake meat" veggie products loaded with additives. They are processed and, unless organic, probably contain genetically modified (GMO) soy.
- Some soy, as long as it is organic, is very beneficial, especially the phytoestrogens that block the excess estrogen. Here are some resources for you to review and explore the benefits of soy: Chris Wark interview with Dr. Kristi Funk: https://www.facebook.com/watch/?v=5260685853981435
- Article from Dr. Josh Axe: https://draxe.com/nutrition/is-soy-bad-for-you

Sodium Chloride
- Commercial table salt is highly processed and full of aluminum, chemicals, and toxic additives. Instead, use a healthier version in moderation, such as pink Himalayan sea salt or Bragg's amino acids.

Aspartame, Sweet 'N Low, Equal, Splenda
- Aspartame is an artificial, chemical sweetener found in many foods and beverages. Words like diet, low sugar, or no sugar added are a good indicator a food probably has an artificial sweetener.
- Another name you will see is sucralose, the generic form of Splenda. These artificial sweeteners may cause cancer or neurological problems, such as dizziness, migraine headaches, weight gain, increased appetite, and bloating.
- In its pure form, Stevia is a healthier alternative to sweeteners. Use in moderation.

Food Colorings (Blue 1, 2; Red 3; Green 3; Yellow 5, 6)
- Six food colorings on the market are linked with cancer in animal testing. There is evidence that food coloring and food additives contribute to behavioral problems in children, and lead to lower IQ, hyperactivity, ADHD, depression, hormonal dysfunction, and cancer. See: https://www.additudemag.com/feed-your-childs-focus-adhd-food-nutrition/

Processed/Refined Wheat and Gluten
- Refined wheat and gluten essentially become like glue while traveling through your intestine, making assimilation of other nutrients difficult and impeding elimination.
- A good alternative to regular bread products is Ezekiel Bread, found in the frozen section of many stores. It still needs to be eaten in moderation if you are healing from cancer. While it does contain some gluten, it is a sprouted whole grain with all of the fiber intact, which helps it travel through the intestines where its nutrients are better absorbed.

Genetically Modified Foods (GMO)
- The genes of these foods have been altered in a lab by scientists and machines. Major offenders are soy, corn, cottonseed, rapeseed (canola), papaya, and beets. Buy organic to avoid GMO's or check for the Non-GMO Certification on any packaged foods.

Caffeine
- Caffeine is believed to increase catecholamines, or stress hormones. The stress response elicits cortisol and increases insulin. Studies have shown that ingesting caffeine actually impairs glucose management and insulin sensitivity for type 2 diabetics. Insulin increases inflammation, which promotes cancer and other diseases. See: https://nutritionj.biomedcentral.com/articles/10.1186/s12937-016-0220-7

Reading Food Labels
- It can be helpful on your health journey to understand how to read food labels and understand what is in your food. Here are some resources to get you started: https://www.ideafit.com/nutrition/cracking-the-code-on-food-and-nutrition-labels/

Good, Better, Best Tips

Introduction for section on Good Better Best:

As each lesson concludes, we want to leave you with an idea(s) for how to implement a suggestion from the lesson in an incremental fashion that meets your needs and abilities. Each lesson will give you ideas that are "Good, Better, and Best".

Good Tips: A perfect way to get started implementing healthier healing options. This tip will be less involved from both a time, energy, effort and financial resources.

Better Tips: This tip will progress you further into implementing the lesson idea. More time and cost may be involved in this step.

Best Tips: When you are ready, this tip will give you ideas to help implement the lesson ideas in a more extensive fashion. This could mean significant investment of time, energy, effort, and financial resources.

LESSON 4:

Vitamin D3 is an essential nutrient that has been shown to improve overall outcomes of cancer patients, possibly reducing advancement of cancer to metastatic disease.

Good: Increase your intake of enhanced vitamin D3 foods, such as organic plant-based milk products.

Better: Take a high dose vitamin D3 supplement to ensure you are increasing your Vitamin D3 levels daily.

Best: Vitamin D is known as the sunshine vitamin. For best improvement of your overall D3 levels, sit in the sun for 15-30 minutes during the mid morning hours.

DISCUSSION QUESTIONS/ACTION STEPS:

1. Are there any supplements on the list you would like to add? You should review your bloodwork and talk to your doctor about what supplements you should take.

   _____
   _____
   _____
   _____

2. What do you foresee being the most challenging in regards to dietary change?

   _____
   _____
   _____
   _____

3. What is a dietary adjustment you have already made?

   _____
   _____
   _____
   _____

4. Name your new goal for this month. Consider some obstacles and who you can ask for support in dealing with them. Tell someone in the group specifically what you want to accomplish and how you plan to do it. Remember, you can go from good, to better and best! You can do this!

   _____
   _____
   _____
   _____

CONNECT:

As a participant in a HealingStrong™ group, you have much to take advantage of in your healing journey. Our meetings are just a part of helping you on a consistent basis. Review these resources for things that can help Rebuild, Renew, and Refresh you all month long!

HealingStrong™ website: http://healingstrong.org
HealingStrong™ Facebook page: http://www.facebook.com/healingstrong/
HealingStrong™ Instagram page: https://www.instagram.com/healingstrongofficial/
HealingStrong™ I AM HealingStrong™ Podcast page: https://healingstrong.org/podcast
HealingStrong™ Start Here: https://healingstrong.org/start-here

Remember: "Fear is detrimental to healing, but affirmations based on God's Word help us replace it with courage and strength."

FIYAA AFFIRMATIONS

I will:

- **Forgive** myself and others.
- **Invite** God into all aspects of my life and healing.
- **Yield** to the needs of my body during this healing season.
- **Accept** my diagnosis and symptoms as temporary.
- **Abandon** negative expectations and think possibilities.

WWW.HEALINGSTRONG.ORG

Being a faith-based organization, we are not only passionate about your present healing journey, but also passionate about your eternal destiny as well. Of course, there will come an end to this life for all of us. We want to make sure that we have shared with you how to know that your eternal destiny is in heaven with our Creator, the One who formed you, loves you, and made a simple way for you to know for certain. If you are not a believer in Jesus Christ and would like to learn more about His saving grace, please see these resources: https://healingstrong.org/refresh

NOTES

Lesson 4: Additional Resources for Further Use

"Iodine Uses: Benefits, Side Effects, Recommendations". *Healthline*. 14 March 2019. Web. <https://www.healthline.com/health/iodine-uses#takeaway>.

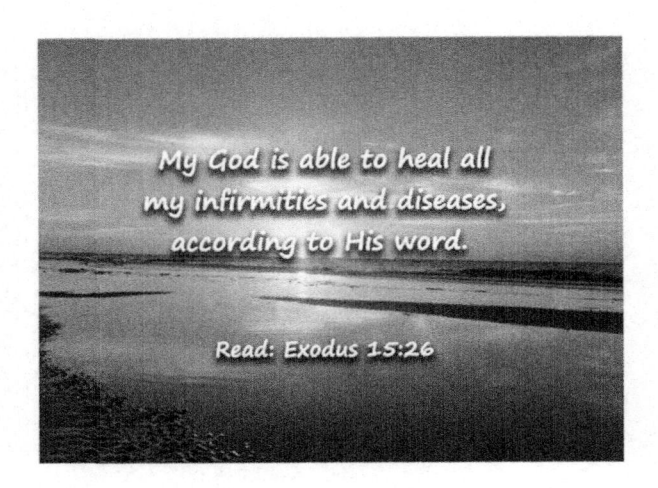

> *My God is able to heal all my infirmities and diseases, according to His word.*
>
> Read: Exodus 15:26

Dear Heavenly Father,

I cry out to You this day, for protection. Guide my steps. Light my path. Make my heart light.

The Spirit we received does not make you slaves, so that you live in fear again; rather, the Spirit you received brought about your adoption to sonship. And by Him we cry, "Abba, Father." The Spirit himself testifies with our spirit that we are God's children.
- **Romans 8:15-16 NIV**

Thank you for your word, Lord. Amen.

Cauliflower Salad
by Bill McCleish

In large bowl, put all together:

- 1 head cauliflower, washed, separated into bite size florets
- 1 green apple, small dice
- 1 cup raw pumpkin seeds
- 1 cup raw cashew pieces
- ½ cup hemp seed

Dressing, mixed in a blender, food processor, etc. Pour over dry ingredients.

- 1/3 cup hemp seed oil
- 1/3 cup flax seed oil
- Juice of 1½ lemons
- 3 dates
- 3 dried figs
- 4 green onions
- 1 teaspoon sea salt

Good source of protein, thiamin, riboflavin, niacin magnesium, phosphorous, dietary fiber, iron, folate, potassium, manganese and copper. Provides Vitamins C, K and B6.

Lesson 5:
7 Steps for Choosing a Non-Toxic Cancer Protocol

> **NOTE:** The full Participant Guide is available for download at our Start Here Page https://healingstrong.org/start-here. Please also review our full disclaimer for HealingStrong™ at: https://healingstrong.org/start-here.

LESSON OBJECTIVE & KEY CONCEPTS

Take Away/Objective:
Choosing and sticking to a non-toxic cancer or healing protocol (either to augment your conventional treatment or on its own) is a serious decision, requiring focus and determination to heal. Prayerfully consider your treatment choice, and then monitor carefully as you journey on your chosen protocol.

Key Concepts:

- Understand the difference between conventional and non-toxic approaches to cancer treatment.
- As you choose your protocol for healing, PRAY continuously for God's direction.
- CHANGE your diet! No matter what treatment route you take, you must support your body with the proper primarily plant-based nutrition.
- Arm yourself with research and knowledge.
- Learn all about your cancer and empower yourself on how to heal it!
- It is helpful and necessary to have an advocate or research partner if choosing alternative therapies.
- Prayerfully choose your protocol then COMMIT to it.
- Monitor yourself carefully and frequently.

DISCUSSION POINTS

***Note to the Reader: Although lessons are geared towards healing from cancer, these lessons are educational in nature and offer information that will equip and empower you with health choices and action steps that you can take that may benefit your overall well-being. If you are on a healing protocol, whether preventative in nature, or treatment that is conventional, holistic or integrative, the principles taught in these lessons may be applied towards a supportive plan for many health challenges.**

"Nature makes the cure; the doctor's job is to aid nature." (Hippocrates, 400 BC)

"The doctor of the future will give no medicine, but will interest his patients in the care of the human frame, in diet, and in the cause, as well as the prevention of disease." (Thomas Edison)

Introduction: Your cancer journey might look something like this: You found a tumor on your body somewhere, but other than that you feel fine. For some of you, you may have had an odd symptom arise, and perhaps your blood work showed evidence of cancer. In either case, what you're realizing is that you have a SYMPTOM of a deeper problem. Your oncologist labels it cancer, because he/she is paid to get rid of cancer. But oncologists rarely discuss how your lifestyle, diet, stress, and other issues have resulted in cancer formation. The progression of this cancer probably took YEARS to reach its current state. Today's lesson empowers you with details of how to manage your cancer.

Conventional treatment of cancer consists of surgery, chemotherapy, radiation, and other pharmaceutical treatments to get rid of the tumor or excess cancer cells. Non-toxic treatments focus primarily on detoxification, nutrition, emotional healing, as well as, vitamin, mineral, enzymatic and herbal supplements to encourage the immune system to heal the cancer. Traditional medical doctors are only taught to treat patients with surgery, chemotherapy and radiation. Alternative therapies are not taught in traditional medical schools. Minimal education on nutrition is required.

In our culture, we have been made to believe cancer (and many other chronic diseases) leaves us helpless and sick. Could it be that much of this fearful belief is painted and enhanced by the side effects and problems resulting from the conventional treatments themselves?

"Once you understand what cancer is, the way it's treated by cancer doctors makes no sense." (Bill Henderson, Cancer Free: Your Guide to Gentle Non-Toxic Healing)

Steps for Choosing a Cancer Healing Protocol
#1 Pray Continuously
#2 Immediately Change Your Diet
#3 Arm Yourself with Research and Knowledge
#4 Learn and Empower Yourself About Your Cancer # 5 Secure an Advocate to Help You
#6 Commit to a Protocol
#7 Monitor Your Progress Frequently

#1 Pray Continuously
Seek God's peace.
The God of peace be with you all. Amen. – Romans 15:33 (NIV)
Peace to the brothers and sisters, and love with faith from God the Father and the Lord Jesus Christ. – Ephesians 6:23 (NIV)

Several things need to be taken into account when deciding which kind of non-toxic cancer protocol is right for you. Prayer is the most important first step to take. If you feel unsettled, don't make a decision. Keep praying. NO cancer type will kill you overnight. In most cases it took YEARS for it to develop to where it is now. If you do have an extremely aggressive cancer, you still have time to seek a second opinion and continue to pray, while you monitor yourself carefully.

When we are placed in a situation that is completely out of our control, who better to be on our side than our powerful Creator? If the body were a building, and it had something terribly wrong with it, wouldn't you want to call on the engineer who designed it? Wherever you are with your spiritual belief and relationship with God, talk to Him about your diagnosis and what to do for treatment. You don't have to tell anyone you're seeking guidance if you're uncomfortable. You have nothing to lose and everything to gain. Look for His promptings, and listen in the quiet moments of prayer for His nudging.

HealingStrong™ offers resources that will help you connect to our Creator and grow in listening to His voice. See: https://healingstrong.org/refresh

#2 Immediately Change Your Diet
Most alternative cancer protocols have diet change of some sort in common. They almost always will focus on organic, raw, plant foods and juicing, so immediately making a change to begin increasing these in your diet is necessary. (See Lesson 3, Cancer Basics and First Steps to Healing and Lesson 4, Helpful Supplements and What Not to Eat When Healing.)

#3 Arm Yourself with Research and Knowledge

The beginning of wisdom is this: Get wisdom. Though it cost all you have, get understanding. – Proverbs 4:7 (NIV)

Begin research on what healing program is best for you. In addition, look up testimonials of people who are living well with what looked like the worst case scenario of the disease. What did they do? HealingStrong™ offers the following resource: Created to Heal Strong by Suzy Griswold. It is a starting point for people wanting to know how they could be open to something that most doctors don't even offer information about in their offices. This is a powerful summary of research by the founder of HealingStrong™ on her journey to discovering alternative strategies by reviewing the:

- Aha! Moment #1: True Healing is Holistic
- Aha! Moment #2: Current Cancer Treatments Aren't Working Well
- Aha! Moment #3: Cancer is a Process, Not a Thing!
- Aha! Moment #4: Sugar Feeds Cancer
- Aha! Moment #5: Oxygen Fights Cancer

The book also includes 14 Testimonials of men and women who have conquered from stage 4 pancreatic cancer, stage 4 melanoma, stage 4 colon cancer, breast cancer, chronic lymphocytic anemia, and other cancers who have incorporated holistic strategies into their protocol. The most powerful part of the book are personally written testimonials provided by: Chris Wark, Ivelisse Page, Bailey O'Brien and many others.

We recommend the book as a starting point for anyone who is even interested in discovering more information about a holistic approach to healing cancer. To access this resource for yourself or your friends or family, go to the HealingStrong™ website: www.healingstrong.org/resources.

Things to know:

- Chemotherapy only has a 2.1% success rate. Chris Wark summarizes in this article: http://www.chrisbeatcancer.com/how-effective-is-chemotherapy/
- Where are the survivors? Arm yourself with testimonials of unexpected survivors. You can find lots of survivor stories that use natural healing. Here are a few sites that offer inspiration:
    - https://healingstrong.org/rebuild
    - http://www.radicalremission.com/index.php/blog
    - http://www.chrisbeatcancer.com/category/natural-survivor-stories/
    - https://cancercompassalternateroute.com/testimonials/
    - https://templetonwellness.com/cancer-survivor-stories/
- One of the best resources available is the DVD Series: Truth About Cancer: A Global Quest. See: https://go.thetruthaboutcancer.com

#4 Learn and Empower Yourself About Your Cancer
- 20 Questions to Ask Your Oncologist was recommended in Lesson 2, Building Confidence: Your Right to Take Charge of Your Health, to help work through the difficult conversation you MUST have, in order to make the best treatment choice for you. You can download the instructions here: https://healingstrong.org/resources
- It is important to know all you can about your disease. Arm yourself with knowledge, but more importantly seek understanding. *The beginning of wisdom is this: Get wisdom. Though it cost all you have, get understanding.* – Proverbs 4:7 (NIV)

#5 Secure an Advocate to Help You
- Make sure your advocate supports your healing choice and will back you up completely. An effective advocate will cheer you on when you want to quit, research for you when you are overwhelmed with a decision, and will tell a critic to give you space.
- An advocate will speak assertively to an overly pushy doctor.
- Pray and ask God to lead you to that person if you cannot think of someone.

#6 Commit to a Protocol

There are many protocols to heal naturally. Prayerfully map out your plan and protocol; then, staunchly dedicate yourself to your healing. No cheating whatsoever. Healing naturally can be overwhelming and expensive. Lesson 6, Healing Protocols and Adjunct Therapies, covers many protocols available. There is a lot of information and plenty of opinions on how to heal. Factors to consider are:

- If you are battling cancer, or any disease - How aggressive is it? How is your current health?
- How much money do you have to spend?
- How much time do you have to commit to healing?
- How driven are you to heal? How much confidence do you have in natural cancer therapies?
- Do you have the support from family and loved ones you need to heal successfully?
- Do you have the resources in your area or the opportunity to move closer to the proper resources that you'll need to heal?

You also need a LONG TERM plan for how you are going to pay for your treatment, which is often out of pocket. Lesson 9, Emotional Healing, discusses how not to go bankrupt in your treatment. Consider your lifestyle and whether you can devote time to natural healing. Lifestyle, travel, support team availability, your age and current health, as well as severity/type of cancer all need to be considered. If you have small children or are caring for an elderly parent, you are going to need additional help! Resources described in Lesson 6, Healing Protocols and Adjunct Therapies, will include, The Gerson Therapy, The Gonzalez Protocol®, Bill Henderson Protocol, Chris Wark's Square One program which can all be used as primary healing protocols.

#7 Monitor Your Progress Frequently

Careful and frequent monitoring of your progress is VERY important when choosing alternative or conventional treatments. You must ensure what you are doing is working. You can review Lesson 2, Building Confidence: Your Right to Take Charge of Your Health, for more details. Along with, or instead of, conventional medical monitoring, these are some options:

HealingStrong's™ Healing Journey Jumpstart video on "How to measure and track your progress through testing: https://healingstrong.org/start-here

Greece Test: Identifies which natural and chemical substances your particular cancer is most sensitive to.

https://breastcancerconquerorshop.com/ product/greece-test/

https://www.rgcc-group.com/tests/

CAProfile: A panel of blood and urine tests compiled by Dr. Emil Schandl.

https://americanmetaboliclaboratories.com/services/

Ultrasound: This looks for blood flow. If you have a tumor, this is a great way to see how effective your treatment is. HerScan is an option for ultrasound for breasts. It is especially good for dense breasts. https://www.herscan.com/

Thermography: Detects changes in the breasts by using surface temperature correlated to blood flow and possible cancer involvement. It examines heat patterns for diagnostics. http://www.breastthermography.com/breast_thermography_mf.htm

Nagalese Blood Test: Nagalase is a protein made by all cancer cells and viruses. This test is an ideal test for monitoring the effect of therapy of cancer and certain viral infections, including HIV & Autism.

https://gcmaf.se/patient-resources/nagalase-blood-test/

Good, Better, Best Tips

Introduction for section on Good Better Best:

As each lesson concludes, we want to leave you with an idea(s) for how to implement a suggestion from the lesson in an incremental fashion that meets your needs and abilities. Each lesson will give you ideas that are "Good, Better, and Best".

Good Tips: A perfect way to get started implementing healthier healing options. This tip will be less involved from both a time, energy, effort and financial resources.

Better Tips: This tip will progress you further into implementing the lesson idea. More time and cost may be involved in this step.

Best Tips: When you are ready, this tip will give you ideas to help implement the lesson ideas in a more extensive fashion. This could mean significant investment of time, energy, effort, and financial resources.

LESSON 5:

Ask God for wisdom in making your choice of protocol. *If any of you lacks wisdom, you should ask God, who gives generously to all without finding fault, and it will be given to you. – James 1:5, NIV*

Good: Implement step #1, Pray continuously. Pray about your choices of protocols. Research your options. Surrender the decision to God. When it is God's will, you will feel at peace about it within your heart. NO MATTER what the many voices around you may be saying, "*Trust in the Lord with all your heart, and do not lean on your own understanding. In all your ways acknowledge him, and he will make straight your paths." Proverbs 3:5-6, NIV*

Better: Implement Step #2, change your diet immediately. Proceed with changing your diet regardless of if you have picked a protocol to use.

Best: Implement Steps 3 and 4. Arm yourself with research and knowledge. Learn and empower yourself about your cancer.

DISCUSSION QUESTIONS/ACTION STEPS:

1. Which of the 7 steps do you feel most confident about? Which is most intimidating to you?

   _____
   _____
   _____
   _____
   _____
   _____
   _____

2. Has anyone present monitored their cancer with any of the mentioned tests? What was your experience?

   _____
   _____
   _____
   _____
   _____
   _____
   _____

3. Can anyone share an example of a story, research study, or survivor that has inspired you on your journey?

   _____
   _____
   _____
   _____
   _____
   _____
   _____

CONNECT:

As a participant in a HealingStrong™ group, you have much to take advantage of in your healing journey. Our meetings are just a part of helping you on a consistent basis. Review these resources for things that can help Rebuild, Renew, and Refresh you all month long!

HealingStrong™ website: http://healingstrong.org
HealingStrong™ Facebook page: http://www.facebook.com/healingstrong/
HealingStrong™ Instagram page: https://www.instagram.com/healingstrongofficial/
HealingStrong™ I AM HealingStrong™ Podcast page: https://healingstrong.org/podcast
HealingStrong™ Start Here: https://healingstrong.org/start-here

Remember: "Fear is detrimental to healing, but affirmations based on God's Word help us replace it with courage and strength."

FIYAA AFFIRMATIONS

I will:

- **Forgive** myself and others.
- **Invite** God into all aspects of my life and healing.
- **Yield** to the needs of my body during this healing season.
- **Accept** my diagnosis and symptoms as temporary.
- **Abandon** negative expectations and think possibilities.

WWW.HEALINGSTRONG.ORG

Being a faith-based organization, we are not only passionate about your present healing journey, but also passionate about your eternal destiny as well. Of course, there will come an end to this life for all of us. We want to make sure that we have shared with you how to know that your eternal destiny is in heaven with our Creator, the One who formed you, loves you, and made a simple way for you to know for certain. If you are not a believer in Jesus Christ and would like to learn more about His saving grace, please see these resources: https://healingstrong.org/refresh

NOTES

Lesson 5 Additional Resources for Further Use

For Additional Support

- https://www.anticancermom.com - Excellent resource on natural healing and simple living
- https://beatcancer.org/ – Excellent resources, Coaching
- https://www.believebig.org/ - Excellent resource for mistletoe therapy and cancer support
- http://www.breastcancerconqueror.com/ - Breast Cancer Conqueror - Dr Veronique Desaulniers
- https://cancercompassalternateroute.com - Good resource for healing cancer with alternative therapies
- https://healingstrong.org - Website has many free resources, blog posts, downloadable materials, a podcast with testimonies, and several HealingStrong™ books including the 30 Day Healthy Living Guide, a daily jumpstart guide, with devotions, recipes and how to do coffee enemas.
- https://templetonwellness.com - Templeton Wellness Foundation is a comprehensive collection of James Templeton's own research and resources to surviving cancer through holistic and alternative medicine.

Resource Clinics

- Linda Isaacs, MD - NYC (Partner of the late Nicholas Gonzalez MD) - http://www.drlindai.com
- Hope 4 Cancer Institute - Tijuana & Cancun, Mexico - Dr. Tony Jiminez - http://www.hope4cancer.com
- Gerson Clinic – Mexico - https://gerson.org/gerpress/gerson-clinic-mexico/
- CHIPSA (Gerson Therapy + adjunct therapies) - Tijuana, Mexico - http://chipsahospital.org
- Hoxsey Bio-Medical Clinic - http://www.hoxseybiomedical.com/ clinic-information/
- North Baja Cancer Clinic - http://www.gersontreatment.com/
- Mistletoe (Integrative) Physicians - https://www.believebig.org/integrative-practitioner/
- An Oasis of Healing - Mesa, AZ —Thomas Lodi, MD - http://www.anoasisofhealing.com
- Forsythe Cancer Care Center - Reno, NV - James Forsythe, MD - http://www.drforsythe.com

"Cancer Tutor: Budwig Therapy". *Cancer Doctor.* 16 Dec. 2015. Web. <http://www.cancertutor.com/budwig>

"Facebook Bill Henderson Online Support Group." *Facebook.* 16 Dec. 2015. Web. <http://www.facebook.com/groups/billhendersonprotocol/>

"The Budwig Protocol "CCFO" - Green Drink Diaries." *Green Drink Diaries.* 26 Jan. 2011. Web. <http://www.anticancermom.com/the-budwig-protocol-ccfo>

> All the battles of my life are the Lord's. As I stand in faith, He fights them for me.
>
> Read 1 Samuel 17:47

Ratatouille
by Sandra Campbell

- 1 Japanese eggplant, slice and salt – let sit 30 minutes – rinse and medium diced
- 1 red bell pepper, medium diced
- 1 medium onion, diced
- 1 zucchini, diced
- 1 yellow squash, diced
- 1 medium tomato, diced
- 1 lemon, very small diced
- 6 cloves of garlic, large chopped

Toss all ingredients with 2 Tablespoons olive oil, season with salt and pepper. Put in a single layer on parchment paper covered sheet pan. Roast 30 minutes 400 degrees.

Rich in Vitamins B6, A, C, E and K. Good source of calcium, selenium, thiamin, folate, potassium, manganese, iron, magnesium, phosphorus, zinc and copper, Contains protein and dietary fiber.

Dear Lord,

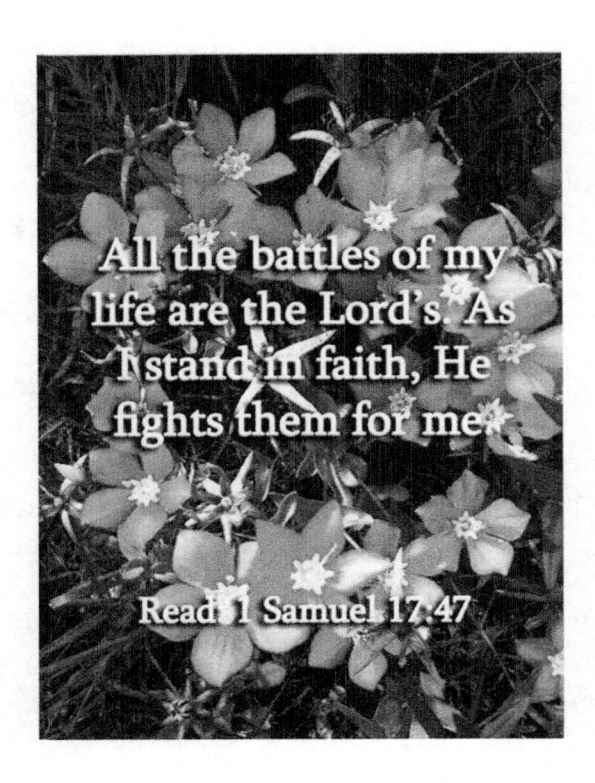

Today, Lord God, I am praying for strength, wisdom and patience. I ask that You give me a clear picture of living my life to the very fullest. I pray that not one day goes by without fully acknowledging that it is a gift, wrapped by You, and that I am not really in control; but that You are!

And the Lord will guide you continually and satisfy your desire in scorched places and make your bones strong; and you shall be like a watered garden, like a spring of water, whose waters do not fail. — Isaiah 58:11 ESV

Thank You for the promises in Your Word. Amen.

Lesson 6:
Healing Protocols and Adjunct Therapies

> **NOTE:** The full Participant Guide is available for download at our Start Here Page https://healingstrong.org/start-here. Please also review our full disclaimer for HealingStrong™ at: https://healingstrong.org/start-here.

LESSON OBJECTIVES & KEY CONCEPTS

Take Away/Objective:

There are hundreds of natural therapies we can use to help aid our bodies in healing from cancer and other health challenges naturally. In this lesson we will look at a few of the more popular complete protocols as well as options that can be used as adjunct therapies.

Key Concepts:

- Many non-toxic cancer protocols address the underlying cause of disease. These protocols can also be used for other chronic issues and health problems.

- The Gerson Therapy, The Gonzalez Protocol®, Bill Henderson Protocol, Chris Wark's Square One program can all be used as primary healing protocols.

- There are also many adjunct therapies that can be combined or used separately as support for healing.

- Cancer clinics both inside and outside the US, along with functional medicine doctors and holistic practitioners, can be an excellent resource for finding care that is right for you.

DISCUSSION POINTS

***Note to the Reader:** Although lessons are geared towards healing from cancer, these lessons are educational in nature and offer information that will equip and empower you with health choices and action steps that you can take that may benefit your overall well-being. If you are on a healing protocol, whether preventative in nature, or treatment that is conventional, holistic or integrative, the principles taught in these lessons may be applied towards a supportive plan for many health challenges.

Introduction: Last meeting we talked about *The 7 steps to Choosing a Healing Protocol*. This week we're going to go into the basics of some of the more popular and successful non-toxic methods for healing.

Basic Description of Specific Cancer Protocols

This is a lesson where you will hear the word cancer a lot. Non-toxic protocols that address cancer, also address other chronic diseases and health problems. If you find a protocol that gets to the root cause of the disease, it will improve overall health and impact and strengthen your immune system. In the book, Cancer: Step Outside the Box, Ty Bollinger details advanced natural cancer protocols and provides a roadmap with discussion of facts and deceptions about cancer and cancer treatments. The best protocols address all aspects of health: diet and nutrition, detoxification, vitamins, minerals, and herbal supplements, as well as emotional and spiritual healing. It may also be necessary to address dental toxins, such as mercury amalgams or root canals. Some specific protocols are listed below with a brief description. While we point out highlights of the protocols, you should research in detail the one you are putting into practice. Other resources may also be found at the end of this lesson.

Chris Wark's Square One Protocol

- Chris Wark created a coaching program for cancer patients, caregivers, and anyone who is serious about prevention called SQUARE ONE. This program is an easier to follow program and contains the specific step-by-step strategies and protocols used by everyone Chris Wark knows who has healed cancer holistically.
- This is the same program that Chris used to heal from his cancer.
- He uses a program of a plant based anti-cancer diet, detoxification, elimination of stress, spiritual healing and forgiveness, exercise, herbs and supplements, and on-going testing. His program is video module based and offers a facebook support group. He offers his program via download and also in DVD and hardcopy.

Resources for Chris Wark's Square One Protocol

- https://healingstrong.org/resources
- https://www.chrisbeatcancer.com
- On Facebook: https://www.facebook.com/groups/squareonesupport/
- *Chris Beat Cancer: A Comprehensive Plan for Healing Naturally* by Chris Wark
- Connect with a HealingStrong™ Group Leader either online or in person. All Group Leaders have access to the Square One Program and can offer a viewing if you are unable to gain access to the program.

The Gerson Therapy™

- The Gerson Therapy™ and diet, created by Dr. Max Gerson in the mid-1900's, is still used successfully today.
- From The Gerson Institute website (see below): "The Gerson Therapy™ is a natural treatment that activates the body's extraordinary ability to heal itself through an organic, plant-based diet, raw juices, coffee enemas and natural supplements."
- In the book, Healing the Gerson Way, Charlotte Gerson (Dr. Gerson's daughter) explains the necessity: "The moment a patient is put on the full therapy, the combined effect of the food, the juices, and the medication causes the immune system to attack and kill tumor tissue, besides working to flush out accumulated toxins from the body tissues. This great clearing-out procedure carries the risk of overburdening and poisoning the liver —the all-important organ of detoxification, which, in a cancer patient, is bound to be already damaged and debilitated."
- Main aspects consist of a vegan diet, Hippocrates Soup (formulated by Hippocrates himself), 10 to 13 vegetable/fruit juice combinations, multiple supplements, and several coffee enemas per day.
- Coffee Enemas were first popularized by Dr. Gerson. Until about 1984, they were listed in the Merck Manual for detoxification and pain relief. Other well-known, pioneering doctors who have suggested use of coffee enemas include: William Donald Kelley, DDS; Harold Manner, PhD.; Dr. Nicholas Gonzales and Dr. Linda Isaacs.
- HealingStrong™ offers webinars with these doctors who discuss the protocols. An example of one of those is Dr. Linda Isaacs webinar: https://vimeo.com/400820159

Resources for The Gerson Therapy™

- Gerson Institute: https://gerson.org
- *Healing the Gerson Way: Defeating Cancer and Other Chronic Diseases* by Charlotte Gerson
- *The Gerson Therapy* by Charlotte Gerson (Handbook can be purchased at https://www.amazon.com/Gerson-Therapy-Nutritional-Program-Illnesses/dp/1575666286)
- On Facebook: https://www.facebook.com/groups/Gersonsupport/
- The Gerson Therapy provides a course to individuals. You can sign up for the course on their website here: https://gerson-institute.teachable.com/
- The Gerson Miracle Movie: https://youtu.be/4SwBpSY2Ymg

The Gonzalez Protocol®
- Embryologist John Beard proposed that proteolytic enzymes make up the body's main defense against cancer. He proposed that enzyme therapy would be an effective cancer defense. He tested his theory, finding that pancreatic enzymes had the ability to dissolve tumors in mice.
- Several decades later, a dentist by the name of Dr. William Kelley used high doses of pancreatic enzymes, a diet high in raw fruits and vegetables, grains and seeds, along with detoxing therapies to cure his own pancreatic cancer. He later changed the approach and introduced metabolic typing, since people have individual diet requirements (either vegan, vegetarian, or carnivorous diets). A gem of a document that is free on the internet that Dr. Kelley wrote regarding his "One Answer to Cancer" can be downloaded here: https://soilandhealth.org/book/dr-kelleys-do-it-yourself-book-one-answer-to-cancer
- Kelley treated thousands of patients successfully on a high dose pancreatic enzyme therapy.
- The late Dr. Nicholas Gonzalez furthered Dr. Kelley's work

Resources for The Gonzalez Protocol®
- The Gonzalez Protocol®: http://cancercompassalternateroute.com/therapies/enzyme-therapy
- *Cancer: Curing the Incurable Without Surgery, Chemotherapy or Radiation* by Dr. William Kelley
- The Nicholas Gonzalez Foundation: https://thegonzalezprotocol.com
- The Gonzalez Protocol® recommended books: www.newspringpress.com

Budwig Protocol
- Dr. Budwig realized that feeding terminal cancer patients an oxygen-rich oil like flaxseed oil partnered with a sulfur-rich protein like quark or cottage cheese, made an obvious and exceptional difference in their health. (Many were brought back to full health). The Budwig mixture is often used in conjunction with other supplemental protocols.
- The diet Dr. Johanna Budwig's created is mostly vegan combined with the "Budwig mixture" of 2/3 cup 1-2% organic cottage cheese (or quark) blended with 6 Tbsp organic flaxseed oil and then mixed with 2 Tbsp of freshly ground flax seeds. When buying whole flax seeds, store in dark place, and grind them fresh. See this article on using and storing flaxseeds: https://cleangreensimple.com/article/does-flaxseed-go-bad/
- This mixture is required several times daily along with additional whole, unadulterated foods.

Resources for the Budwig Protocol
- Cancer Doctor: https://cancerdoctor.com/treatment/budwig/
- Anti-Cancer mom Description and Personal Testimonial: https://www.anticancermom.com/the-budwig-protocol-ccfo/#more-164
- *The Budwig Cancer & Coronary Heart Disease Prevention Diet: The Complete Recipes, Updated Research & Protocols for Health & Healing* by Johanna Budwig
- A Day in the Budwig Diet: Learn Dr. Budwig's Complete Home Healing Protocol Against Cancer, Arthritis, Heart Disease and More (DVD and/or book) by Ursula Escher

Bill Henderson Protocol
- According to the book, *Cancer-Free: Your Guide to Gentle Non-Toxic Healing*, this protocol modifies and supplements Dr. Budwig's protocol, including a once daily serving of the cottage cheese and flaxseed oil mixture.
- Other primary elements are: a mostly raw, organic, vegan diet of salads, smoothies and juices, as well as reduced fruit intake. No processed foods of any kind are allowed, including sugar, meat, and dairy (with the exception of cottage cheese, which loses its dairy properties when blended with flaxseed oil).
- Caffeine is limited to green tea. Various supplements Bill Henderson recommends include the immune system booster, Transfer Point Beta 1, 3D Glucan.
- This protocol is an excellent base, which can be supplemented with adjunct therapies listed below or used with other protocols with very little interference. It is also less labor intensive than Gerson or the complete Budwig Protocol and more affordable than most others.
- Note: some people may have sensitivities to the large amount of oil in the Budwig mixture or with the taste. Also, in rare cases, the dairy may cause lactose sensitivity, so the Bill Henderson Protocol can help avoid these issues.

Resources for Bill Henderson Protocol
- *Cancer-Free: Your Guide to Gentle, Non-toxic Healing* by Bill Henderson
- Complete Explanation of the Bill Henderson Protocol: http://www.anticancermom.com/how-i-beat-cancer
- On Facebook: www.facebook.com/groups/billhendersonprotocol/

Adjunct Therapies
Adhering to your primary protocol is important for long-term success. Adjunct therapies may be used to maximize the primary therapy's effectiveness.

Essiac Tea
- Immune boosting and detoxing tea used for cancer patients.
- Watch documentary: https://genuineessiac.com/pages/see-how-rene-caisse-a-canadian-nurse-brought-essiac-tea-into-the-mainstream-in-this-video
- See the details of the herbs in the tea in this article, and about use and easy preparation: www.anticancermom.com/essiac

Beta-1, 3D Glucan
- As seen above in the Bill Henderson Protocol and Lesson 4, Helpful Supplements and What Not to Eat When Healing, this supplement helps the immune system identify cancer cells. It is taken daily, 30 minutes before food.
http://www.anticancermom.com/beta-1-3-d-glucan/

Essential Oils
- Essential oils are plant-based, God-given medicine, which have been used since the dawn of time. If you were to search in PubMed for various essential oils and their effectiveness with disease, you may be surprised! For example, with peppermint oil alone, there are 1,000 published scientific studies.
- Two good resources on Essential Oils are: Dr. Z's (Eric Zielinski, D.C.) website https://naturallivingfamily.com/ and Dr. Z's book *The Healing Power of Essential Oils*.
- Frankincense oil is one of the most powerful essential oils to use when healing. See: https://draxe.com/essential-oils/what-is-frankincense/   https://naturallivingfamily.com/frankincense-essential-oil-benefits

Supplements
- Selenium, vitamin D, magnesium, high dose vitamin C, iodine, and a high dose multivitamin are among the most common vitamin and mineral deficiencies. (See Lesson 4, Helpful Supplements and What Not to Eat When Healing, for additional information.)

Turmeric/Curcumin
- There are more scientific articles written about curcumin in fighting cancer than any other supplement. See: https://www.chrisbeatcancer.com/four-cancer-fighting-spices/ https://www.ncbi.nlm.nih.gov/pmc/articles/PMC7446227/

Cannabis Oil
- Cannabidoiol (CBD) is extracted from the hemp plant and legal in 50 states.
- Purity and potency should be tested both for effectiveness and legal limits of THC, which meet each state's standards. In PubMed, there are over 1,500 peer-reviewed studies on CBD, showing strong evidence to support its useful impact on dozens of diseases, including cancer. See: www.projectcbd.org

Hyperthermia Therapy
- This treatment increases the body temperature to a level where it starts killing or destabilizing cancer cells. See: https://hope4cancer.com/alternative-cancer-treatments/full-body-hyperthermia/
https://www.cancer.gov/about-cancer/treatment/types/hyperthermia

Hyperbaric Therapy
- Hyperbaric Oxygen Therapy (HBOT) is breathing 100% oxygen while under increased atmospheric pressure.
- Articles on hyperbaric therapy can be found at: http://hyperbaricphp.com/studies-articles/ https://www.ncbi.nlm.nih.gov/pmc/articles/PMC3510426/

Fasting
- Fasting restricts calorie intake, starving cancer cells while protecting healthy cells. It is common to fast in conjunction with hyperbaric and hyperthermic therapy. See: https://restorativemedicine.org/journal/intermittent-fasting-cancer/ https://www.chrisbeatcancer.com/the-fast-lane-to-health/ https://healingstrong.org/rebuild
- Oxygen and water are the most important nutrients for the human body. Thus, water plays an important metabolic role in all functions in the body. Water fasting is an important tool that can be used to boost immunity and health. Fasting is a process that may help to boost the body's ability to heal. Water fasting before chemotherapy has been proven to be protective of healthy cells. Dr. Valter Longo of University Southern California has offered insight on this topic. In addition, short and long-term water fasting is a way to destroy unhealthy cells and reset metabolism. There are clinics that are available to support long-term fasts. A HealingStrong™ webinar about this topic can be seen here by Dr. Anja Sonst: https://vimeo.com/661074270/876d05ce85.
- Dr. Tony Jimenez has a video on non-water fasting available for review here: https://vimeo.com/321970955/644c228564

B-17/ Laetrile/ Amygdalin
- Apricot and apple seeds contain a controversial vitamin that has been shown to fight cancer cells. B-17 or Laetrile (chemical name) is taken either orally or intravenously and has properties that slows down the spread of illness in the body, including cancer. One theory reported in International journal of Radiation and Biology (https://www.ncbi.nlm.nih.gov/books/NBK65988/) is that the B17 may help increase the production of pancreatic enzymes, which is important for fighting cancer cells. (Dr. Linda Isaacs, MD - https://vimeo.com/400820159)
- Another article detailing these seeds is here: https://draxe.com/nutrition/apricot-seeds/
- A great documentary about the history behind this cancer fighter is Apricot Kernels and Laetrile: https://www.youtube.com/watch?v=tPADSv3XAv0

Ozone Therapy
- Ozone therapy has been utilized and studied for many decades. Its effects are proven, consistent and with minimal side effects.
- Many practitioners are using ozone therapy to increase the amount of oxygen in the body. It heals and detoxifies the body at the same time. For more information about Ozone Therapy: https://cancerdoctor.com/treatment/ozone-therapy/

High Dose Vitamin C
- Chris Wark notes "High dose vitamin C is a powerful anti-viral, anti-bacterial, and anti-cancer protocol."
- https://www.chrisbeatcancer.com/high-dose-vitamin-c-protocol-for-cancer/
- https://cancercompassalternateroute.com/antioxidants-vitamins-and-minerals/vitamin-c-therapy/

For Additional Support
- https://www.anticancermom.com - Excellent resource on natural healing and simple living
- https://beatcancer.org/ – Excellent resources, Coaching
- https://www.believebig.org/ - Excellent resource for mistletoe therapy and cancer support
- http://www.breastcancerconqueror.com/ - Breast Cancer Conqueror - Dr Veronique Desaulniers
- https://cancercompassalternateroute.com - Good resource for healing cancer with alternative therapies
- https://healingstrong.org - Website has many free resources, blog posts, downloadable materials, a podcast with testimonies, and several HealingStrong™ books including the 30 Day Healthy Living Guide, a daily jumpstart guide, with devotions, recipes and how to do coffee enemas.
- https://templetonwellness.com - Templeton Wellness Foundation is a comprehensive collection of James Templeton's own research and resources to surviving cancer through holistic and alternative medicine.

Resource Clinics

- Linda Isaacs, MD - NYC (Partner of the late Nicholas Gonzalez MD) - http://www.drlindai.com
- Hope 4 Cancer Institute - Tijuana & Cancun, Mexico - Dr. Tony Jiminez - http://www.hope4cancer.com
- Gerson Clinic – Mexico - https://gerson.org/gerpress/gerson-clinic-mexico/
- CHIPSA (Gerson Therapy + adjunct therapies) - Tijuana, Mexico - http://chipsahospital.org
- Hoxsey Bio-Medical Clinic - http://www.hoxseybiomedical.com/clinic-information/
- North Baja Cancer Clinic - http://www.gersontreatment.com/
- Mistletoe (Integrative) Physicians - https://www.believebig.org/integrative-practitioner/
- An Oasis of Healing - Mesa, AZ —Thomas Lodi, MD - http://www.anoasisofhealing.com
- Forsythe Cancer Care Center - Reno, NV - James Forsythe, MD - http://www.drforsythe.com

Good, Better, Best Tips

Introduction for section on Good Better Best:

As each lesson concludes, we want to leave you with an idea(s) for how to implement a suggestion from the lesson in an incremental fashion that meets your needs and abilities. Each lesson will give you ideas that are "Good, Better, and Best".

Good Tips: A perfect way to get started implementing healthier healing options. This tip will be less involved from both a time, energy, effort and financial resources.

Better Tips: This tip will progress you further into implementing the lesson idea. More time and cost may be involved in this step.

Best Tips: When you are ready, this tip will give you ideas to help implement the lesson ideas in a more extensive fashion. This could mean significant investment of time, energy, effort, and financial resources.

LESSON 6:

Choose a protocol. CHOOSE LIFE! CHOOSE TO SEE YOURSELF WHOLE AND HEALED. *I have set before you life and death, blessing and curse; therefore choose life, that you and your offspring may live. Deuteronomy 30:19 ESV*

Good: Review your options for protocols outlined in this lesson. Commit to a protocol.

Better: Find a support group for your protocol. Many are listed in the lesson. Join a group for support! Many groups will answer all your questions as you begin to implement your chosen protocol.

Best: Choose an adjunct therapy to go along with your protocol. Begin to implement it!

DISCUSSION QUESTIONS/ACTION STEPS:

1. Do you feel peace in regards to your route to healing? If so, what does peace feel like to you, mentally, spiritually and physically? How did you arrive at your decision?

   _____
   _____
   _____
   _____
   _____
   _____
   _____

2. What kind of support do you need on your healing journey?

   _____
   _____
   _____
   _____
   _____
   _____
   _____

3. What is your goal for this month? What are some obstacles? Tell someone in the group what you want to accomplish and how you plan to do it.

   _____
   _____
   _____
   _____
   _____
   _____
   _____

CONNECT:

As a participant in a HealingStrong™ group, you have much to take advantage of in your healing journey. Our meetings are just a part of helping you on a consistent basis. Review these resources for things that can help Rebuild, Renew, and Refresh you all month long!

HealingStrong™ website: http://healingstrong.org
HealingStrong™ Facebook page: http://www.facebook.com/healingstrong/
HealingStrong™ Instagram page: https://www.instagram.com/healingstrongofficial/
HealingStrong™ I AM HealingStrong™ Podcast page: https://healingstrong.org/podcast
HealingStrong™ Start Here: https://healingstrong.org/start-here

Remember: "Fear is detrimental to healing, but affirmations based on God's Word help us replace it with courage and strength."

FIYAA AFFIRMATIONS

I will:

- **Forgive** myself and others.
- **Invite** God into all aspects of my life and healing.
- **Yield** to the needs of my body during this healing season.
- **Accept** my diagnosis and symptoms as temporary.
- **Abandon** negative expectations and think possibilities.

WWW.HEALINGSTRONG.ORG

Being a faith-based organization, we are not only passionate about your present healing journey, but also passionate about your eternal destiny as well. Of course, there will come an end to this life for all of us. We want to make sure that we have shared with you how to know that your eternal destiny is in heaven with our Creator, the One who formed you, loves you, and made a simple way for you to know for certain. If you are not a believer in Jesus Christ and would like to learn more about His saving grace, please see these resources: https://healingstrong.org/refresh

NOTES

Lesson 6 Additional Resources for Further Use

Bollinger, Ty M. *Cancer: Step Outside the Box. 2nd ed.* McKinney, TX: Infinity 510^2 Partners, 2007. Print.

Frahm, Anne E., and David J. Frahm. *Cancer Battle Plan: Six Strategies for Beating Cancer From a Recovered "Hopeless Case"* Colorado Springs, Colo.: Pinþ on. 1992. Print.

"Patent US6630507 - Cannabinoids as Antioxidants and Neuroprotectants."

Aidan Hampson-Julius Axelrod-Maurizio Grimaldi- The United States Of America As Represented By The Department Of Health And Human Services - https://www.google.com/patents/US6630507

Somers, Suzanne. *Knockout: Interviews with Doctors Who Are Curing Cancer-and How to Prevent Getting It in the First Place.* New York: Crown, 2009. Print.

The Beautiful Truth: The World's Simplest Cure for Cancer - DVD (available on Amazon for purchase)

"Testimonials of Healing Cancer Naturally." Cancer Compass An Alternate Route. 17 Dec. 2015. Web. <http://cancercompassalternateroute.com/testimonials/>.

"The Incredible Story of Laetrile." *The Truth About Cancer.* Nair, Suresh. 4 Sept 2021. <https://thetruthaboutcancer.com/search/Laetrile/>

"VICTORY OVER CANCER." VICTORY OVER CANCER. 16 Dec. 2015. Web. <http://www.drkelley.info/>

> God holds me in His hands. He makes me strong so I am not afraid.
>
> Read: Isaiah 41:10

healingstrong

Green Smoothie
by Cortney Campbell

- 4 cups filtered water
- 1 cup filtered ice
- ½ avocado (no pit!)
- 3 handfuls of baby greens, spinach
- 1 cup broccoli sprouts
- 1 handful of sunflower sprouts or buckwheat lettuce sprouts
- ½ any color pepper
- 1 medium tomato
- 2 whole carrots (even the leafy tops are really good!)
- 1 cup lentil or mung bean, sprouted for 2 days (if I don't have these I will add cooked black beans.)
- 1 apple (cut in 8 pieces)

Put in blender and blend well.

Other additions or substitutes: cilantro, cucumber, 1 cup raw broccoli, cayenne pepper, oregano, coconut oil, or anything else raw, healthy and organic you want to try in this green concoction.

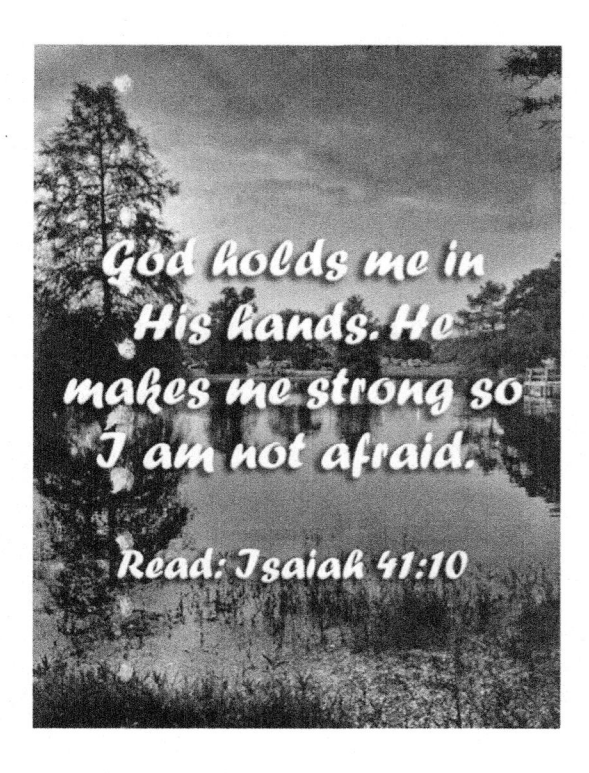

Dear Lord,

Whether you turn to the right or to the left, your ears will hear a voice behind you, saying, "This is the way; walk in it."- Isaiah 30:21 NIV

Lord, I pray that I always walk in Your unfailing light and that I always hear Your words. Guide my steps so that I may reflect the light, Your light within me.

Thank you for the promises in Your Word. Amen.

Lesson 7:
Basics on Toxins and Why We Need to Detox to Heal

NOTE: The full Participant Guide is available for download at our Start Here Page https://healingstrong.org/start-here. Please also review our full disclaimer for HealingStrong™ at: https://healingstrong.org/start-here.

LESSON OBJECTIVES & KEY CONCEPTS

Take Away/Objective:

Knowledge is power. In order to effectively heal the body of any ailment or disease, we must recognize and address the toxic threats we are exposed to everyday.

Key Concepts:

- Understand toxins in our food, and potential risks of commonly used products, and contaminants in our air and water.

- Identify and discuss healthier alternatives that we can use in our daily living.

- Understand your body's natural detox route, including first and second lines of defense functions.

DISCUSSION POINTS

***Note to the Reader: Although lessons are geared towards healing from cancer, these lessons are educational in nature and offer information that will equip and empower you with health choices and action steps that you can take that may benefit your overall well-being. If you are on a healing protocol, whether preventative in nature, or treatment that is conventional, holistic or integrative, the principles taught in these lessons may be applied towards a supportive plan for many health challenges.

Understanding Toxins

In order to understand the value of a lesson on detoxing, it is important that you first realize how the body works as a defense mechanism against toxins.

- A breakdown in our health (sickness or disease) means our defense mechanism is compromised.
- Toxic buildup in the body is much like garbage overflow in a dump. If it sticks around long enough, predators, varmints, and other disease-causing culprits attack.
- Toxin comes from a Greek word meaning arrow dipped in poison. Toxins include: bacteria, viruses, parasites, fungi, and environmental toxins such as pesticides, food additives, refined sugars, preservatives, and plastics are pathogenic and make us sick.
- External toxins are coming at us in all directions and undermine our health. Once inside our body, these contaminants can attack vital organs including the heart, liver and kidneys.
- Our drinking water, our food, the air we breathe, the products we put on our skin, the mattresses we sleep on, even the water we shower or bathe in are full of toxic chemicals.
- Since World War II, over 80,000 chemicals have entered daily use. Four billion pounds of chemicals are released by American industries yearly. See https://www.ecowatch.com/battle-lines-are-drawn-as-congress-reforms-the-40-year-old-toxic-subst-1882175722.html.
- Per an article by the Environmental Working Group (EWG) nearly all of us have the chemicals PFOA or PFOS in our bloodstream. These are chemicals that are now banned in the United States, but manufacturers are still creating similar chemicals. We once saw these chemicals in the form of Teflon and 3M Scotchgard. These chemicals have been linked to cancer and kidney disease. A Canadian study indicates that 90% of umbilical cords tested have these chemicals as they are being transmitted from mother to child. See https://www.ewg.org/news-insights/news/childrens-exposure-pfas-chemicals-begins-womb.

Once toxins enter our body, a healthy immune system will deal with them. However, when a person is dealing with cancer or other chronic health issues, TOXINS WILL UNDERMINE THE IMMUNE SYSTEM'S ABILITY TO EFFECTIVELY HEAL.

Where are the most common toxins found and what can be done?

Food

Problem: If your food comes from a box, bag or can, it typically has toxic chemicals in it. Stabilizers, flavor preservatives, colors and dyes are all additives or preservatives. Diet products containing artificial sweeteners are highly toxic. There are thousands of GRAS or Generally Recognized As Safe chemicals and additives, which are not required to be listed on food labels by the Food and Drug Administration (FDA). So, what is in our food?

Solution: Eat whole (unprocessed) foods: organic, non-GMO (genetically modified) fruits and vegetables when possible. Green, leafy vegetables are detoxifying. If you choose to eat meat or fish, eat grass fed, hormone and antibiotic-free beef, as well as free-range, non-GMO fed chicken and fish. And avoid these fish due to high levels of toxins: Bluefin Tuna, Chilean Sea Bass, Grouper, Orange Roughy, Swordfish and Yellow Perch to name a few. See https://seafood.edf.org/guide/worst.

Plastics

Problem: According to the FDA, plastics are called food contact substances, but until April 2002, they were referred to as indirect food additives. The new name (of course) removes the implication that plastic gets into your food. Phthalates are used in plastic bottles, plastic wrap, and many plastic toys. Many plastics also contain BPA and flame retardants. As plastic breaks down, it can absorb other toxins more easily, such as damaging pesticides like DDT, PCB and PAH. Plastic is found in canned goods, as well. Look for cans that are BPA free. Many cans are coated with a thin layer of plastic on the inside of the can, directly contacting your food. Toxins found in plastics are stored in our fat cells.

Solution: Limit or eliminate your plastic use, especially during healing. Do not eat foods that have been stored or heated in plastic containers. Use a glass mason jar or stainless steel bottle instead of drinking from plastic water bottles. If you need to buy plastic items, make sure they do not contain BPA. Look for the recycling codes 1, 2, and 5 on the bottom of the container, since they are less likely to contain BPA and other phthalates. Never microwave your food in plastic containers or wash plastic in the dishwasher. Heating up plastic causes the toxins to leach or seep out of the container and into your food or drink. Instead, heat in glass and ceramics and eliminate use of the microwave! Heating in a convection oven only takes a few more minutes than a microwave. See http://www.niehs.nih.gov/health/materials/endocrine_disruptors_508.pdf.

Microplastics

Problem: Microplastics are pieces of plastic less than 5 millimeters long created by the breakdown process. They can enter the bloodstream and go into our cells. People are ingesting the equivalent of a credit card weekly! These are found in seafood, bottled water, tap water, salts, alcohol, clothing and exfoliants for your skin. See https://www.healthline.com/health-news/how-dangerous-are-microplastics-to-your-health.

Solution: We need to communicate through how we spend our money. As much as possible, buy products that do not contain plastic. Also, talk to your representatives about incentives for manufacturers to create plastic products that will break down sooner.

Tap Water

Problem: Drinking tap water can be detrimental to your health. Heavy metals, chemicals, and bacteria can contaminate our water supply along with remnants of prescription drugs that have been flushed down the toilet. Fluoride and chlorine are also a concern, which is covered in Lesson 11, Dental Toxins.

Solution: Humans are predominantly composed of water (about 66 percent by weight for men and about 60 percent for women). The amount of water we consume is critical to effectively and efficiently flush toxins out of our systems. The average person should drink at least eight 8-ounce glasses of filtered water a day. However some protocols incorporate extensive juicing and advise you focus on drinking juices and less on drinking water. You can check on the quality of your tap water at https://www.ewg.org/tapwater/. An effective water filter is important. A reverse osmosis water filtration system is the best for removing most chemicals, bacteria, and other toxins. It also helps to install water filters on bathroom faucets, as well. A shower filter is a good place to start. A Natural News independent study found Berkey to be #1 in filtration effectiveness (http://www.waterfilterlabs.com/). As an affiliate, when you shop Berkey on https://healingstrong.org/resources you help support the mission of HealingStrong™. The most popular water filters for removal of toxic heavy metals such as lead, cadmium, mercury, arsenic, and elements with radioactive isotopes uranium, strontium, cesium) were independently tested, and Berkey was most effective.

Air

Problem: Toxins in the air come from asbestos that could be in older buildings, our polluted, smoggy city air, and moldy and chemical-laden household environments.

Solution: Avoid exercising outside on busy streets, especially during rush hour. Rural areas are not as much of a risk. A good practice is to check the air quality real-time using https://www.airnow.gov/. Air purifiers with HEPA and UV filter technology can help indoors. If an air purifier is not in your budget, change your heating/cooling system filters often and open your windows to air out your house before allergy season begins. Whether you're at the nail salon, mechanic shop, paint store, bars, or just standing on the side of the road, if you smell chemicals, they are entering your body. Avoid being in these situations for long periods of time, but if you must, wear a mask with an effective filtering system.

Body Care and Cleaning Products

Problem: According to the EWG, almost 89% of the 10,500 known cosmetics and skin care ingredients have not been evaluated for safety by the Cosmetic Ingredient Review, the FDA or any other publicly accountable institution per https://www.ewg.org/news-insights/statement/fda-warns-cosmetics-industry-follow-law-untested-ingredients. The American government does not require health studies or pre-market testing of chemicals in personal care products, even though we are exposed to them. Most shampoo, face wash, deodorant, lotion, diaper rash cream, laundry detergent, toothpaste, fingernail polish, hair color, hairsprays, colognes, and perfumes contain toxic chemicals. Even some products labeled natural and/or organic may contain chemically-derived additives, which are generally recognized as safe and not legally required to be listed on the label.

Solution: Choose everyday products without petroleum, phosphates, aluminum, mineral oil, paraffin, sulfates, chlorine, ammonia, and artificial fragrance. Products contained in biodegradable, BPA-free, packaging are available online, if not in local stores. Visit the EWG's website at http://www.ewg.org and search for your products in its comprehensive guides (healthy cleaning, sunscreens, cosmetics and other skincare products). Most deodorants and antiperspirants contain aluminum, which can be harmful to the lymph nodes. (Easy deodorant recipe: http://www.anticancermom.com/homemade-coconut-oil-deodorant/).

The Body's First Line of Attack – OUTERMOST GUARDS

Your first line of defense includes physical and natural chemical barriers, which are prepared to defend the body. These include the skin, tears, mucus, cilia, stomach acid, urine flow, and friendly gut bacteria.

Skin

Skin is the body's largest organ, which uses its water repellent mechanisms to keep bacteria at bay. However, constant use of chemicals breaks down this natural barrier.

Tears, Mucus, Saliva and Perspiration

Your nose, mouth, and eyes are obvious entry points for toxins. Tears, mucus, and saliva protect the eyes, nose, and throat by providing lubrication, cleansing and protection. Sweating is also the immune system's way of ridding our bodies of toxins.

Suppressing tears increases stress levels, and contributes to diseases such as high blood pressure, heart problems and peptic ulcers, which commonly precede cancer. A build-up of chemicals in the body due to mental stress are removed by tears. Toxic thoughts create chemical reactions within our bodies that can pollute our immune systems. (https://answersingenesis.org/human-body/the-miracle-of-tears/)

Cilia

Cilia are very fine hairs lining the windpipe, which move mucus and trapped toxic particles away from the lungs.

Stomach Acid
Stomach acid kills bacteria and parasites that have been ingested; however, it does not deactivate toxins. Rather, toxins actually deactivate stomach acid, causing digestive issues.

Urine Flow
Urine flow flushes out toxins from the bladder area.

Friendly Gut Bacteria
You have beneficial bacteria growing on your skin, in your bowel and other places in the body such as the mouth and the gut. If it is compromised, the body's ability to heal is compromised. A damaged gut wall allows overgrowth of bad bacteria, parasites, and fungus, causing chronic inflammation related to bloating, constipation, and intestinal pain.

The Body's Second Line of Attack – INNERMOST GUARDS
The second line of defense is the immune system, a group of cells, tissues and organs working together to protect the body.

Army of Cells
We have an army of cells that include: Neutrophils, T Helper and T Killer Cells, Macrophages, Dendritic Cells, B Cells, and Suppressor T Cells. This army of cells is first on scene, cleaning up dead cells and searching for any foreign substance, which slows down the body's defense mechanisms. This innate part of our immune system destroys invading microorganisms. (https://www.niaid.nih.gov/research/immune-cells)

The Lymph System
The lymphatic system fights off infections, parasites and abnormal cell growth like cancer. As long as it is functioning in peak condition, it will filter out toxins and bodily invaders. However, if the lymphatic system is burdened by a poor diet, lack of exercise, lingering viruses, and excess toxins, it cannot eliminate them. The body then begins to show symptoms of disease. Unlike many of the other systems in the body, the lymph system does not have a pump to transport its fluid. Instead, it relies on physical exercise to move lymph fluid throughout the body. The less we move, the weaker our immune systems become.

Liver and Kidneys
The liver works like a factory and is the primary organ in the body to safely remove toxins from the blood. Cells in the liver convert a fat soluble toxin to a less harmful water soluble one or package them for easier disposal through the bile or urine. The kidneys are responsible for flushing waste from the blood.

In Lesson 8, Strategies to Detox, we will discuss strategies to detox.

Good, Better, Best Tips

Introduction for section on Good Better Best:
As each lesson concludes, we want to leave you with an idea(s) for how to implement a suggestion from the lesson in an incremental fashion that meets your needs and abilities. Each lesson will give you ideas that are "Good, Better, and Best".

Good Tips: A perfect way to get started implementing healthier healing options. This tip will be less involved from both a time, energy, effort and financial resources.

Better Tips: This tip will progress you further into implementing the lesson idea. More time and cost may be involved in this step.

Best Tips: When you are ready, this tip will give you ideas to help implement the lesson ideas in a more extensive fashion. This could mean significant investment of time, energy, effort, and financial resources.

LESSON 7:

The most common environmental toxins known to weaken our immune systems include: Glyphosate, Mold & Mycotoxins, Phthalates, Heavy Metals, Organophosphates, Xylene and Microbial Endotoxins. Learn where these toxins are found and make changes to begin eliminating them from your daily routine.

Good: Inventory and replace your personal hygiene products, household cleaning agents, lawn care products, pantry shelf items with items that are SAFE, CLEAN and free of toxins. Begin by replacing one or two items at a time as they empty.

Better: Make your own personal care and home cleaning products. Most items can be easily made with safe and effective everyday ingredients. By mixing your own, you'll not only save money, but be ensured of quality and no hidden ingredients.

Best: While eliminating the toxins from your daily routine, begin taking measures to cleanse the toxins from your body by drinking half your body weight in ounces of water, eat an immune boosting/anti-oxidant/anti-inflammatory diet, include fasting in your protocol and supplements that support your liver in detoxification as well as rebounding or other daily movement and exercise.

DISCUSSION QUESTIONS/ACTION STEPS:

1. In which areas of your life do you recognize the need to reduce your exposure to toxins?

   _____
   _____
   _____
   _____
   _____
   _____
   _____

2. Which toxins are the most difficult to stay away from? Which are the sneakiest?

   _____
   _____
   _____
   _____
   _____
   _____
   _____

3. What strategies will you use to reduce your exposure to toxins?

   _____
   _____
   _____
   _____
   _____
   _____
   _____

CONNECT:

As a participant in a HealingStrong™ group, you have much to take advantage of in your healing journey. Our meetings are just a part of helping you on a consistent basis. Review these resources for things that can help Rebuild, Renew, and Refresh you all month long!

HealingStrong™ website: http://healingstrong.org
HealingStrong™ Facebook page: http://www.facebook.com/healingstrong/
HealingStrong™ Instagram page: https://www.instagram.com/healingstrongofficial/
HealingStrong™ I AM HealingStrong™ Podcast page: https://healingstrong.org/podcast
HealingStrong™ Start Here: https://healingstrong.org/start-here

Remember: "Fear is detrimental to healing, but affirmations based on God's Word help us replace it with courage and strength."

FIYAA AFFIRMATIONS

I will:

- **Forgive** myself and others.
- **Invite** God into all aspects of my life and healing.
- **Yield** to the needs of my body during this healing season.
- **Accept** my diagnosis and symptoms as temporary.
- **Abandon** negative expectations and think possibilities.

WWW.HEALINGSTRONG.ORG

Being a faith-based organization, we are not only passionate about your present healing journey, but also passionate about your eternal destiny as well. Of course, there will come an end to this life for all of us. We want to make sure that we have shared with you how to know that your eternal destiny is in heaven with our Creator, the One who formed you, loves you, and made a simple way for you to know for certain. If you are not a believer in Jesus Christ and would like to learn more about His saving grace, please see these resources: https://healingstrong.org/refresh

NOTES

Lesson 7 Additional Resources for Further Use

"10 toxic chemicals to avoid in personal care products." *NaturalHealth365 Powerful Solutions.* Lori Alton. 15 June 2019. Web. <https://www.naturalhealth365.com/toxic-chemicals-3012.html>

"Baby care products: possible sources of infant phthalate exposure." *PubMed.* Sathyanarayana S, Karr CJ, Lozano P, Brown E, Calafat AM, Liu F, Swan SH. Feb 2008. Web. <http://www.ncbi.nlm.nih.gov/pubmed/18245401>.

"Decrease in anogenital distance among male infants with prenatal phthalate exposure." *PubMed.* Swan SH, Main KM, Liu F, et al. Aug 2005. Web. <http://www.ncbi.nlm.nih.gov/pubmed/16079079>.

"Detoxify your Life Series, Part I: Introduction and Baby Products." *MyKidHasCancer.com.* 18 Aug 2015. Web. <https://thesternmethod.com/detoxify-your-life-series-part-i-introduction-and-baby-products/>.

"Detoxify Your Life Series, Part II: Safe Personal Care Products." *MyKidHasCancer.com.* 19 Aug 2015. Web. <https://thesternmethod.com/detoxify-your-life-series-part-ii-personal-care-products/>.

"Detoxify Your Life Series, Part III: Cleaning Products." *MyKidHasCancer.com.* 28 Aug. 2015. Web. <https://thesternmethod.com/detoxify-your-life-series-part-iii-cleaning-products/>.

"The Pollution in People." *EWG.* 24 June 2016. Web. <https://www.ewg.org/research/pollution-people>.

"Remove Dangerous Chemicals From Your Personal Care Routines." *BWellBHealthy.com.* 10 Apr 2017. Web. <https://bwellbhealthy.com/2017-3-4-b40uo7ph7u11mbfs64lqcc5qk5q64i/>.

"Synthetic Polymer Contamination in Bottled Water." *PubMed.* Mason, Sherri A.; Welch, Victoria G.; Neratko, Joseph. 11 Sep 2018. Web. <https://www.ncbi.nlm.nih.gov/pmc/articles/PMC6141690/>.

Somers, Suzanne. **TOX-SICK: How Toxins Accumulate to Make You Ill—and Doctors Who Show You How to Get Better.** Harmony. 19 April 2016. Print.

"Unsafe Ingredients." *Cosmetic Ingredient Review.* 2016. Web. <https://www.cir-safety.org/supplementaldoc/unsafe-ingredients>.

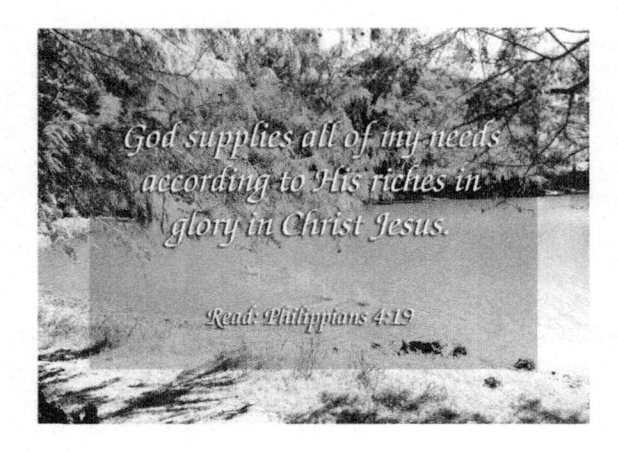

God supplies all of my needs according to His riches in glory in Christ Jesus.

Read: Philippians 4:19

Dear Heavenly Father,

Thank you for Your presence in my life.

Where can I go from Your Spirit? Where can I flee from Your presence? If I go up to the heavens, You are there;

If I make my bed in the depths, You are there.

If I rise on the wings of the dawn, if I settle on the far side of the sea, even there Your hand will guide me, Your right hand will hold me fast. **-Psalm 139:7-10 NIV**

Thank you for your word, Lord. Amen.

Chopped Kale Salad

- ½ bunch kale - any variety
- 1 large carrot - organic - peeled and cut into ribbons with vegetable peeler
- 1 small red bell pepper, chopped
- ½ avocado - pitted and cut into small chunks
- 1 Tablespoon chopped sweet onion
- handful basil, chopped
- handful cilantro, chopped

Dressing
- ¼ cup avocado oil
- 2 Tablespoons rice vinegar
- 1 Tablespoon grated ginger
- 1 Tablespoon Tamari
- 1 teaspoon lime juice
- 1 garlic clove, minced
- 1 Tablespoon toasted pine nuts

Take out rough stems from kale, chop leaves coarsely, put in a large bowl and then sprinkle with Himalayan sea salt, massage salt into kale. Let rest 5 minutes. Add the rest of ingredients to the bowl and toss together.

Whisk dressing ingredients together and toss with salad.

Lesson 8:
Strategies to Detox

> **NOTE:** The full Participant Guide is available for download at our Start Here Page https://healingstrong.org/start-here. Please also review our full disclaimer for HealingStrong™ at: https://healingstrong.org/start-here.

LESSON OBJECTIVE & KEY CONCEPTS

Take Away/Objective:
Taking charge of our health and making appropriate changes will help the body heal strong. There are many ways to help our body to cleanse and detoxify itself.

Key Concepts:

- Educate yourself on strategies available to deep cleanse and help heal your body from the toxic load.
- Identify toxic thought patterns in your life. These lead to chemical responses in the body that are detrimental towards healing.

DISCUSSION POINTS

***Note to the Reader: Although lessons are geared towards healing from cancer, these lessons are educational in nature and offer information that will equip and empower you with health choices and action steps that you can take that may benefit your overall well-being. If you are on a healing protocol, whether preventative in nature, or treatment that is conventional, holistic or integrative, the principles taught in these lessons may be applied towards a supportive plan for many health challenges.

Introduction: At our last meeting we talked about WHY detoxification is important in healing, so this week we are going to talk about HOW we do it. At the end of our meeting I'd love to hear ways detoxification has personally worked for you and how you've found time to work it into your week.

When diagnosed with a major illness, it can be difficult or even impossible to pinpoint the cause. Detoxification is vital and eliminates a variety of potential culprits.

Rebounding
- Rebounding is done on a high-quality mini-trampoline. Exercise aids the detoxification process, but jumping on a rebounder defies gravity to pump the cells and help cleanse the lymph system.
- The lymph system relies on physical exercise to move lymph fluid throughout the body.

Colon Cleanses
- The body absorbs nutrients and pollutants accumulate in the colon, so regular elimination two to three times a day is an important part of healing.
- A toilet stool can help put you in the proper position for easier elimination.
- Hydro-Colon Therapy is a process in which warm water is flushed through the colon (via your rectum) in order to safely clean your large intestine. Colonics are typically administered by a licensed colon hydrotherapist.

Enemas and Liver Cleanse
- Coffee enemas cleanse the liver, rather than the colon, by stimulating the body's production of glutathione, theobromine, and theophylline.
- The caffeine, theobromine and theophylline, in coffee dilate the ducts to facilitate bile flow. The palmitates in coffee increase the action of glutathione-S-transferase by 600% to 700% in the liver and in the small intestine. It is this enzyme that is responsible for the detoxification of free radicals and it's also this enzyme that inhibits the reabsorption of the toxic bile. The quart of fluid held in the colon encourages the bowels to quickly move the waste out of the body by increasing peristalsis. https://naturalnews.com/026289_coffee_coffee_enemas_coffee_enema.html
- A good guide for how to do a coffee enema can be found here: https://thehealthyfamilyandhome.com/detox-and-cleanse it-kits/coffee-enemas/.
- A great resource provided by Chris Wark is a video with Dr. Vickers discussing the benefits of coffee enemas and it can be viewed here: http://www.chrisbeatcancer.com/dr-vickers-explains-coffee-enemas-for-healing-cancer/
- HealingStrong™ offers a *30 Day Healthy Living Guide,* available to all Members in the Member's Lounge, provides extensive details about why the coffee enema is beneficial and a step-by-step instruction guide. https://healingstrong.org/resources.
- It is important to note that if you are a chemotherapy patient, then detoxifying the liver needs to be done gradually after all chemotherapy has been stopped. Chemotherapy works in conflict with detoxifying the liver.

Connection by Suzy

As a holistic cancer thriver, the one part of the Gerson protocol I had the most trouble with was the coffee enemas. It took me six months into a holistic protocol to warm up to the idea of doing the enemas. My health mentor and friend, Wendy Hood, came over one morning and asked me why I was "sitting on the enema bucket? She gave me a swift "kick" in my pride, and encouraged me to heal strong. It wasn't until I incorporated the enemas into my daily routine that I began to see drastic improvement in my overall health and reduction in tumors. I actually look forward to them today and use the time to listen to and meditate on scriptures using an app on my phone. This is a great way to schedule quiet time as everyone will leave you alone when you are doing a coffee enema! Coffee enemas are powerful. Don't shy away from them.

Liver and Gallbladder Cleanse
- Another way to detoxify is through a liver and gallbladder cleanse. A liver and gallbladder cleanse can assist in eliminating any gallstones that have developed over time in your body. A healthy liver and gallbladder will aid in improved overall health. In the book by Andreas Moritz "The Amazing Liver and Gallbladder Flush" he describes a procedure for doing a liver and gallbladder cleanse. Several flushes are required over several months to clear the gallbladder and liver of gallstones.

Parasite Cleansing
- Most people have some type of parasite living in our bodies. When the immune system is compromised, these can wreak havoc on the body. Pumpkin seeds, hot peppers, and herbal remedies are all used as treatments. Black walnut hull tincture combined with ground cloves and wormwood has proven effective in cleansing parasites. (http://www.naturalnews.com/037964_parasites_detox_cleanse.html)

Dry Brushing
- Dry brushing helps to rid the body of trapped toxins and even unclogs pores. Using repetitive strokes towards the heart with a non-synthetic brush stimulates the lymphatic system and exfoliates the skin. To see how, watch Cancer Rehab PT's video: https://www.youtube.com/watch?v=1YnVb9le-r0.

Oil Pulling
- Oil pulling is an ancient Ayurvedic dental technique, which draws out toxins and improves oral health by swishing coconut oil in the mouth on an empty stomach for around 20 minutes and then releasing it into a plastic cup that you will throw away when full. Do not swallow. It may even whiten teeth! To see how, watch Dr. Axe's video: https://www.youtube.com/watch?v=DtFzd3TBYil.

Chlorella
- This green algae is a powerful heavy metal detoxifier. If you have a mouth full of amalgams ("silver" or mercury fillings), chlorella is an important daily supplement. According to Natural News, chlorella is a chelating agent, or a substance that binds with heavy metal toxins. In turn, this makes it easier for the body to expel heavy metals. (https://naturalnews.com/2018-02-15-four-science-backed-benefits-of-chlorella.html)

Turmeric and Curcumin
- This spice helps protect against environmental mutagens. Curcumin is a product of turmeric and has excellent healing properties. A study at India's Panjab University found that curcumin inhibited mutations by as much as 80% against all mutagens tested in foods. (http://www.lifeextension.com/Magazine/2005/9/cover_dna/Page-01)

Vitamin C
- Also known as ascorbic acid, this is a water-soluble nutrient and antioxidant found in some foods and is important for cellular growth and repair. You cannot overdose. Too much Vitamin C causes diarrhea or bowel upset. Reduce the level of Vitamin C until you find your tolerance. https://draxe.com/nutrition/best-vitamin-c-supplement-benefits.
- Choose one that contains piperine and dihydroquercetin for better synthesis in the body. https://www.lifeextension.com/magazine/2013/5/a-better-form-of-vitamin-c.
- A Vitamin C flush is something to consider doing if you have been exposed to a lot of environmental toxins, you are sick with a virus, or you just need a boost to your immune system. For how to do this flush see: https://www.fxmedicine.com.au/blog-post/naturopathic-vitamin-c-flush.

Milk Thistle Extract
- This is an herb that's been used for thousands of years to support liver, kidney, and gallbladder health. It contains the flavonoid silymarin, which is thought to be responsible for many of its beneficial effects, including liver protection and antioxidant, anti-viral, and anti-inflammatory properties.

Green Tea and White Tea
- These herbs have powerful antioxidants called catechins and flavonols. The extract from the tea prevents DNA damage, triggers DNA repair mechanisms and also helps detoxify the liver.

Iodine
- Thanks to environmental pollutants, iodine deficiency has become a worldwide epidemic. In the book, The Iodine Crisis, author Lynne Farrow discusses the importance of iodine supplementation in healing. Iodine displaces fluoride from the thyroid receptors, along with bromide and chelates all of the heavy metals to begin removing them from the body. There is a protocol behind it, which includes other supplements for support, but iodine is the key. Iodine is important for every cell in the body.

Chanca Piedra
- This is an herb that is widely used around the world to support the urinary tract. It's nickname is stone breaker, as it has acclaim for breaking up kidney stones. Here is an article to read more about this very powerful detoxifying herbal remedy: https://www.verywellhealth.com/chanca-piedra-4799790.

Juicing
- Juicing aids detoxification and floods the body with nutrients. Devote 3 to 14 days (or more for an advanced juice fast) to consuming only raw, fresh, organic, vegetable and fruit juices. Kale, swiss chard, celery, cucumber, beet, carrot, lettuce, ginger, and lemon are all excellent choices for increasing nutrient levels (buying bottled juice is not sufficient). Once the juice fast is finished, continue juicing every day to maintain nutrient balance and aid detoxification. The Gerson protocol, in addition to many others, uses extensive juicing as the foundation for treating disease.
- Two juicing documentaries we recommend are Jason Vale's Super Juice Me (https://www.youtube.com/watch?v=Aaxa7rxEbyk) and Joe Cross in Fat, Sick and Nearly Dead (https://vimeo.com/147549662).
- In addition, Juice Lady Cherie provides extensive detox and juicing recipes at www.juiceladycherie.com. Her five-day raw foods and juicing retreats are very popular to help others get a jumpstart on detoxing. Cherie also put together some slides for HealingStrong™ called Juicing Your Way to Health, which are presented here by a group leader: https://healingstrong.org/start-here.

Detox the Mind
- The Bible has a lot to say about detoxing our mind. How we perceive ourselves and others has a direct impact on our health. Taking every thought captive for Christ is important to our well-being. (See 2 Cor.10:5)

Good, Better, Best Tips

Introduction for section on Good Better Best:

As each lesson concludes, we want to leave you with an idea(s) for how to implement a suggestion from the lesson in an incremental fashion that meets your needs and abilities. Each lesson will give you ideas that are "Good, Better, and Best".

Good Tips: A perfect way to get started implementing healthier healing options. This tip will be less involved from both a time, energy, effort and financial resources.

Better Tips: This tip will progress you further into implementing the lesson idea. More time and cost may be involved in this step.

Best Tips: When you are ready, this tip will give you ideas to help implement the lesson ideas in a more extensive fashion. This could mean significant investment of time, energy, effort, and financial resources.

LESSON 8:

Start implementing detox routines into your daily schedule.

Good: Begin intentional lymphatic drainage every morning through a simple practice of dry brushing before you shower or as part of your morning routine. It's an easy way to begin stimulating your lymph nodes.

Better: Engage in daily exercise like walking, swimming, dancing, rebounding. Get the blood moving.

Best: Try your first coffee enema and add to your routine.

Discussion Questions/Action Steps:

1. Have you ever experienced any of the detoxification protocols we talked about today?

2. Are you interested in trying any of the detoxification strategies we discussed today?

3. What steps are you going to take to incorporate detox strategies into your daily routine?

4. Will you commit to detoxing those things that have infected your mind?

CONNECT:

As a participant in a HealingStrong™ group, you have much to take advantage of in your healing journey. Our meetings are just a part of helping you on a consistent basis. Review these resources for things that can help Rebuild, Renew, and Refresh you all month long!

HealingStrong™ website: http://healingstrong.org
HealingStrong™ Facebook page: http://www.facebook.com/healingstrong/
HealingStrong™ Instagram page: https://www.instagram.com/healingstrongofficial/
HealingStrong™ I AM HealingStrong™ Podcast page: https://healingstrong.org/podcast
HealingStrong™ Start Here: https://healingstrong.org/start-here

Remember: "Fear is detrimental to healing, but affirmations based on God's Word help us replace it with courage and strength."

FIYAA AFFIRMATIONS

I will:

- **Forgive** myself and others.
- **Invite** God into all aspects of my life and healing.
- **Yield** to the needs of my body during this healing season.
- **Accept** my diagnosis and symptoms as temporary.
- **Abandon** negative expectations and think possibilities.

WWW.HEALINGSTRONG.ORG

Being a faith-based organization, we are not only passionate about your present healing journey, but also passionate about your eternal destiny as well. Of course, there will come an end to this life for all of us. We want to make sure that we have shared with you how to know that your eternal destiny is in heaven with our Creator, the One who formed you, loves you, and made a simple way for you to know for certain. If you are not a believer in Jesus Christ and would like to learn more about His saving grace, please see these resources: https://healingstrong.org/refresh

NOTES

Lesson 8 Additional Resources For Further Use

"7 Methods for Detoxing and Cleansing Your Body of Toxins." *Natural Society.* 22 Feb. 2022. Web. <http://naturalsociety.com/7-methods-holistic-detox-cleansing-body-toxic-exposure/ #ixzz3bMdS3xgn>

"10 toxic chemicals to avoid in personal care products." *NaturalHealth365 Powerful Solutions. Lori Alton.* 15 June 2019. Web. <https://www.naturalhealth365.com/toxic-chemicals-3012.html>

"Best Intermittent Fasting Strategies & Hot to Fast." *Dr. David Jockers.* Web. <https://drjockers.com/best-intermittent-fasting-strategies/>.

Calbom, Cherie and Calbom, John. **Juicing, Fasting and Detoxing for Life: Unleash the Healing Power of Fresh Juices and Cleaning Diets**. Grand Central Life & Style. 2014. Print.

Farrow, Lynne, and David Brownstein. **The Iodine Crisis: What You Don't Know About Iodine Can Wreck Your Life.** Devon Press. 2013. Print.

Gerson, Charlotte. **The Gerson Therapy**. Kensington. 2001. Print.

"Micronutrient Information Center." *Selenium.* June 2015. Web. <http://lpi.oregonstate.edu/mic/minerals/selenium>

Morse, N.D., Robert. **The Detox Miracle Sourcebook E-Book.** Kalindi Press. 11 Sept. 2013. Print.

> *I will fix my thoughts on what is true, and HONORABLE, and right, and PURE, and lovely, and admirable. Think about things that are excellent and worthy of praise.*
>
> Read: Phillippians 4:8

Coconut Energy Balls

- ½ cup coconut oil
- ½ cup maple syrup
- ½ cup raw organic cacao powder
- 2 cups raw, chopped nuts of your choosing - Soaked overnight and then dehydrated
  (I use a cashew - pecan combo most of the time but walnuts and almonds are also great)
- 2 Tablespoons raw pumpkin seeds, coarsely chopped
- 1 teaspoon chia seeds
- 1 cup raw, unsweetened coconut

Mix together coconut oil, maple syrup and cacao powder until thoroughly blended. Add in remaining ingredients and mix well. Form into small balls and freeze. Enjoy cold or thawed.

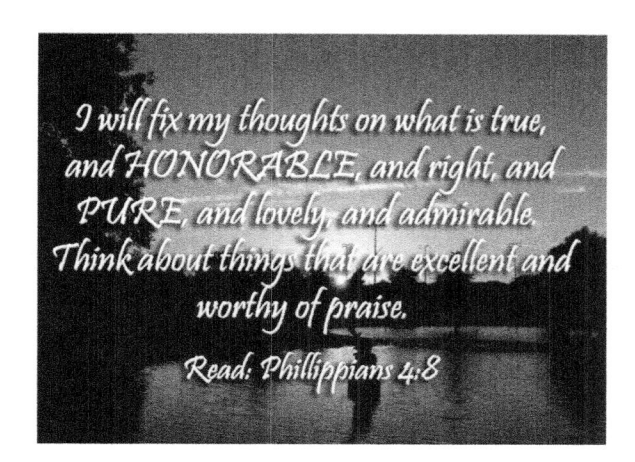

Dear Heavenly Father,

Dear Lord, Emanuel, be with me today. Love and lift me in Your unfailing grace. The battle is a giant, but just as David's faith slew Goliath with a single stone, so too we focus our faith for their battle. Give me the strength, oh, Lord, to slay a giant.

I pray Isaiah 40:31 (NIV) : But those who hope in the Lord will renew their strength. They will soar on wings like eagles, They will run and not grow weary, They will walk and not be faint.

Thank you for Your Word, Lord. Amen.

DISCUSSION POINTS

***Note to the Reader: Although lessons are geared towards healing from cancer, these lessons are educational in nature and offer information that will equip and empower you with health choices and action steps that you can take that may benefit your overall well-being. If you are on a healing protocol, whether preventative in nature, or treatment that is conventional, holistic or integrative, the principles taught in these lessons may be applied towards a supportive plan for many health challenges.**

It is well-accepted in even the medical community that emotional stress can have a negative impact on our health. The mind-body connection is being increasingly confirmed as more and more research is recognizing that the mind and body affect one another in powerful ways.

- Forgiveness has a role to play in our overall health and well-being. Research shows that when we address unforgiveness and emotional stressors physical healing can follow. Holding on to negative emotions with the mind can manifest physically in the form of illness.
- Stressful reactions cause release of inflammation producing hormones, such as adrenaline and cortisol. If this happens often, our bodies become off-balance and illness can take the shape of heart disease, cancer, diabetes, or other chronic illness.
- Stress can be caused by external and internal factors, and is often in response to a situation that feels out of control. However, the one thing we can control is how we respond.

Forgiveness helps our overall state of health - physical, mental and emotional per: https://www.takingcharge.csh.umn.edu/how-do-thoughts-and-emotions-affect-health.
- 70% reported a decrease in their feelings of hurt
- 13% experienced reduced anger
- 27% experienced fewer physical complaints (for example, pain, gastrointestinal upset, dizziness, etc.)

In other studies, practicing gratitude also has an important role to play in our overall state of joy. Dr. Brené Brown has found that there is a relationship between joy and gratitude. Her research reinforced this concept: It's not joy that makes us grateful, but gratitude that makes us joyful. A great short video of Dr. Brown discussing her findings are here: https://www.youtube.com/watch?v=2IjSHUc7TXM&t=157s

***As we run through this list today, jot down notes about where you find yourself with each one. You can even give yourself a rating with "1" being that you are unaffected by this stressor and "10" being that you are greatly affected by this stressor.

Stress from Unforgiveness of Others

This is first on our list because it runs deep and is spiritual at its root.

A heart at peace gives life to the body, but envy rots the bones. Proverbs 14:30 (NIV)

Who is a God like you, who pardons sin and forgives the transgression of the remnant of his inheritance? You do not stay angry forever but delight to show mercy. You will again have compassion on us; you will tread our sins underfoot and hurl all our iniquities into the depths of the sea. Micah 7:18-19 (NIV)

The person being hurt by unforgiveness is the one who won't let go of an offense or wrong. Unforgiveness traps negative energy in your body as you continue to hold onto grudges. This negativity spreads to all parts of your soul (mind, will and emotions), including your self-esteem and expectations. Remember how we discussed the effect of your outlook on your healing? Don't allow an issue from your past to rob you of your well-being today.

We often have to turn to God over and over again in order to be fully set free from the hurts and wrongs in our past. He is the only one who can make old things new, and He loves you enough to desire that you live without the burden of unforgiveness. Forgiveness is not saying that the experience that hurt you is okay. It is saying that you trust God enough to release the person who has wronged you to Him, and that you believe He can heal you from your old wounds. It's important to note that someone holding onto resentment buys into the lie that they are affecting the other person - that somehow the other person is punished because you haven't forgiven them yet. But is that really the case? Are they suffering because of the anger you are holding onto? What does God's Word tell us about forgiving others? We all want to be forgiven, but when it comes time for us to forgive, oftentimes that is a very different narrative.

Choose today to let go of bitterness, resentment, jealousy, grudges, vengeance, and all other negativity fueled by unforgiveness. Grow and move on from it, trusting God to heal former wrongs with His affirming love. How many of our old hurts stem from feeling rejected? Jesus never rejects you. He chooses you today and when we accept His love and forgiveness, we are a new creation. He keeps no record of our wrongs, nor does He hold our sin against us. He forgives our sins. He covers our sins. He remembers our sins no more. (Ps 51:2, Jn 1:9, Ps 32:1,5, Rm 4:7, Isa 43:25, Jer 31:34) That's news I think many of us need to be reminded of today. Allow His deep, abiding love to define your worth rather than a memory from your past. Mentally visualize what your life would be like if you put your old self behind you and walk away from it. Can you see it in the distance becoming smaller and smaller?
Does it feel light? What does that release you to walk towards? Can you see yourself moving towards wholeness and the one true Healer?

Notes:

_____

_____

_____

Stress from Unforgiveness of Self

Subtle beliefs about who we are and whether we are good enough can affect our health. Are you satisfied with where you are in life? Do you tell yourself that you "should" be doing something else, making more money, living somewhere different, being more involved with a particular family member or cause, or doing a better job? Do you beat yourself up about it, or rehearse the ways you don't measure up over and over in your head?

This may sound silly, but sometimes you just need to stop everything and give yourself a big hug. Better yet, give yourself grace. *Hebrews 4:16 (NIV)* reminds us to *"Let us then approach God's throne of grace with confidence, so that we may receive mercy and find grace to help us in our time of need."* Jesus offers that to us. In *Ephesians 2:8 (NIV) - "For it is by grace you have been saved, through faith - and this is not from yourselves, it is the gift of God."* We can never DO enough to earn His love or grace. It is a free gift. When we accept Jesus' gift on the cross, He forgives us and scripture tells us that He remembers our sins (past, present and future) no more. That is good news! (See: Hebrews 10:17) You are a loved child of God and His desire is for us to draw near to Him with confidence and His grace, which is His gift to us through his son, Christ Jesus. (See: Romans 3:24) We've all failed our own expectations, or felt ashamed that we don't measure up to someone else's plan for us. Unconditional love is your birthright won through Jesus' death on the cross. Jesus paid the ultimate price for us and it's only because of Him, nothing we have done or haven't done, that we will ever earn His favor or achieve His righteousness. *"Only in the Lord, it shall be said of me, are righteousness and strength;..." Isaiah 45:24 (ESV).* That's good news! If Jesus forgives us, then let's forgive ourselves.

Do you have questions about God's grace and what He offers you through Jesus? Can we pray with you or for you? Please feel free to email our prayer team and we have an assigned prayer team member every day of the week who will answer you. We also have volunteer chaplains who are available to answer any questions you might have. Your group leader can offer a couple of resources for support in this area: RAK Ministries, or Journey U Ministries.. Please email HealingStrong™ at: prayerrequest@healingstrong.org. If you are not a believer in Christ and would like to learn more about His saving grace, please see these resources: https://healingstrong.org/refresh.

Affirmations are sayings that should be repeated daily, especially when negative feelings arise. With practice and repetition, they can help you reframe your mindset, replacing your old views about yourself and others. Some great affirmations based on scriptures for healing our mind and soul are listed below:
- God goes before me and will see me through this day. Based on Deut. 31:8
- I am a child of the one true God who sees me and loves me. Based on Gen 16:13 and Psalm 82:6
- I am awesomely and wonderfully made. Based on Psalm 139:14
- Today is the day God made and I will choose joy and be glad in it. Based on Psalm 118:64
- Even if others abandon me, the Lord will hold me close. Based on Psalm 27:10

You can find 101 scripture affirmations about healing at https://www.divinerevelations.info/pdf/bible_scriptures_on_healing_3.pdf

Do you have any favorite affirmations you are currently using? Feel free to write it below and keep it close by to refer to it until it becomes part of your self-talk and daily reminders.

Notes:
_____
_____
_____

Stress from Illness

It is empowering to know that even when dealing with stress from illness, there are steps we can take to lessen the effects.

- We can eat to boost our immune system, reduce inflammation, and heal our cells.
- We can take supplements we know will help.
- We can savor the moments that are important to us - a beautiful view, or the touch of a loved one.
- We can research a doctor we trust that will help us learn about our condition and options to help our bodies heal naturally.
- Participants at our meetings are knowledgeable and helpful, too! By being present in your HealingStrong™ group, you are moving towards health and seeking your wellness.
- Tomorrow is out of our control, but today, we make the best choices we can, so that we can walk into tomorrow with contentment that we have done what is possible towards good outcomes, resting in faith for tomorrow.
- We have to let go of other distractions and fears about the future, and let our focus be to connect with our Creator through prayer and trust in His will for us. It's hard to understand, but even our momentary suffering has a purpose. *"For our light and momentary troubles are achieving for us an eternal glory that far outweighs them all."* – 2 Cor. 4:17 (NIV)

Remember, we can reframe "illness" into opportunities. Examples of that are listed below.

- ACCEPT your symptoms as teachable clues rather than fear inducing "problems." Releasing the fear and embracing yourself in the state that you are in right now sends signals to your body that it's going to be OK.
- ACCEPT that you are doing the best you can with the time you have. We've been learning so many things that we could do to improve our health. It is not possible to do them all!
- ACCEPT that you did the best you could with what you knew in the past. It's not healthy to regret decisions we made in the past.
- ACCEPT and love yourself unconditionally, thought by thought. We can learn to be content in the NOW, and release future outcomes.

"Therefore do not worry about tomorrow, for tomorrow will worry about itself. Each day has enough trouble of its own." - Matthew 6:34 (NIV)

Notes:
_____
_____
_____

Stress from Lack of Self Care

Your season of healing is a time to majorly downshift and prioritize your commitments. It is YOUR time to focus on YOU and the energy it will take for you to heal. This will seem unrealistic or even impossible to some of you, but how badly do you want to get well? Changes will need to be made.

- People will need to be asked to help, even those who may not be eager at first.
- Children will need to be given more responsibility and less enabling.
- Spouses will need to take on roles they're not used to.
- Jobs may need to be quit, or a leave of absence taken.

Some of these changes will be really tough, but there is always a solution somewhere. For some of you, the hardest thing to do is accept help, but now is the time. This is a season of healing and now more than ever, a time to pray and ask God for His guidance. Then, walk by faith, not in fear, with Him.

Notes:
_____
_____
_____

Stress from our Jobs and Finances

Too much work, too little work, difficult bosses, annoying co-workers, long commutes, pay cuts and freezes, a job you don't even enjoy - all of this can be VERY distracting! Now is the time to re- evaluate whether the stress from your work is worth your health. Major changes may need to be made, but what is the payoff? Possibly your health and life?

- Consider a temporary leave of absence to give you time to focus on healing.
- Is there a work from home option?
- Get creative and talk with your employer after explaining your situation.

Healing using natural therapies can be a financial concern because of the cost. Setting up an online fundraising account (example: GiveSendGo, or Go Fund Me), discussing financial options with a skilled advisor, or talking with close loved ones about how to address your financial needs should be discussed early in your healing protocol. Minimize the financial burden with a good plan, staying flexible and responsive as needs arise. Your focus does not need to be on your finances; it needs to be on getting well.

We do not believe God intended for you to go bankrupt to heal!

Notes:

_____
_____
_____

Stress from Family and Concerned Family Members

Consider keeping boundaries between you and worrisome or negative loved ones during your healing. If anyone in your life is causing you unnecessary concern, it must be addressed and the issues need to be resolved as best as possible. Even a well-meaning loved one can feel like a drain when you suddenly need to help them process THEIR emotions about YOUR illness.

It is helpful to have an advocate at your side as a buffer so that your full energy can go towards healing. You, or your advocate can tell the curious that you have researched your healing choice, discussed it with your doctor and decided on a course of action. Remember, boundaries between you and others can be helpful for you as you and your Heavenly Father determine what is the best course of action. Your times of rest need to be protected as well, so give yourself permission to be unavailable, if that is best for you during a taxing time. Encourage well-wishers to send uplifting messages in your preferred methods of communication - text, email, Facebook, or even good old fashioned letters! Then they can send their love, while keeping their distance.

Also, if there are people in your life that continue to cause relational drama or tend to evoke emotions of anger or guilt, they need to be kept at a distance as well. Make it right with them and then focus on healing. Being firm and assertive without getting overly dramatic is helpful here. You should never feel guilty about focusing on your health and how YOU feel called to heal! This is also where an advocate or healing partner can be involved and very helpful. A very important part of the healing process is standing firm in your decisions, and moving forward in a spirit of faith. God will guide you, and He will also help you deal with the fall-out.

Reducing Stress through Prayer

Prayer is powerful and an important tool that God has given us. If you haven't been a prayerful person before, there is no better time like the present to begin. Consider seeking out a prayer partner or prayer counselor as a resource for your healing, especially if you are struggling to resolve emotional issues, feeling overwhelmed, or seem to be returning to the same difficulties and problems. Check out HealingStrong™'s Refresh tools (https://healingstrong.org/refresh) to draw closer to God and seek His wisdom in your journey to heal.

Inner healing prayer is also a way to step into wholeness and freedom. There are trained prayer programs that do this, and HealingStrong™ has worked with RAK Ministries (www.rakministry.com) and www.JourneyU.org. Christian Healing Ministries (www.christianhealingmin.org) is also a training organization for those interested in further training in this area. If you are a member of a Bible believing church, ask the leadership to help you find a prayerful member who may be willing to come alongside you and help you walk this journey in prayer. Oftentimes, churches will have a prayer team, prayer service, or someone you can reach out to for added reinforcement. There is a wonderful story in Daniel 10 that highlights when Daniel set his heart and mind to pray and fast, a spiritual battle ensued and this passage shows us the power of praying and fasting…..the angel armies in heaven get to work!

Ask God to guide you towards someone that can pray with you, and for you, as part of your healing team. We all have moments when another's faith can help boost our own.

A favorite story in the Bible is found in Mark 9: Some friends brought their paralyzed friend to Jesus. They interrupted Him as he was speaking to a large group by digging a hole out of the ceiling and lowering their friend right in front of Jesus. Jesus looked up, and it says "Jesus saw their faith", and because of the friends' faith, Jesus healed the man. It's a beautiful reminder of leaning on one another.

Notes:

_____

_____

_____

Recommended Coping Strategies/Practical Skills
1. Forgiveness - If you are carrying around unforgiveness, there is free help:
    - Journey U Ministries: https://www.journeyu.org
    - Rak Ministry: https://www.rakministry.com/ (setup a one on one session, or join an online webinar)
2. Intentional Breathing - We will cover this more in Lesson 12, Sleep, Meditation, and Breathing. Dr. Chatterjee suggests to breathe in three seconds, hold four seconds, and exhale five seconds.
    - "Ocean Breathing" Heals Emotional Pain." http://www.ideafit.com/fitness-library/ldquoocean-breathingrdquo-heals-emotional-pain
    - Malaysia, From. "Do Abdominal Breathing." http://www.wikihow.com/Do-Abdominal-Breathing
3. Positive Thought Dialogue - Dr. Caroline Leaf: Healthy Thoughts vs. Toxic Thoughts - https://www.youtube.com/watch?v=Nrcntl7Jsm0
4. Affirmations - The ones covered here and/or the affirmations Healing Strong shares with every lesson.
5. Possibilities Thinking - The Perfect Attitude to Healing Cancer Successfully: https://www.youtube.com/watch?v=Ozhhg5t76F0.
6. Emotional Freedom Technique
    - Desaulniers, Dr. Veronique. "EFT For Breast Cancer Tutorial." https://www.youtube.com/watch?v=wkxvpN2WtuA.
    - Desaulniers, Dr. Veronique. "How Emotional Freedom Technique Can Help You Fight Cancer." https://thetruthaboutcancer.com/emotional-freedom-technique-cancer/.
    - The Christian Meditator uses EFT for Emotional Pain: https://www.youtube.com/watch?v=VKL1ie27BzQ.
    - "The Tapping Solution (EFT): How To Get Started." http://www.thetapping-solution.com/.
7. Cognitive Behavior Therapy - See: https://www.medicalnewstoday.com/articles/296579#what-can-cbt-treat.
8. Laughter - *"A cheerful heart is good medicine, but a crushed spirit dries up the bones." Proverbs 17:22 (NIV)*
    - The Comedy Cures Foundation. https://www.comedycures.org/laughline.
    - Liebertz, Charmaine. "A Healthy Laugh." https://www.scientificamerican.com/article/a-healthy-laugh/.
    - Victoria Vogt "Can laughter cure illness?" https://science.howstuffworks.com/life/inside-the-mind/emotions/laughter-cure-illness.htm.
9. Journaling - See: https://www.healthline.com/health/benefits-of-gratitude-practice.
10. Christian Counseling or Therapy - To find a local Christian Counselor, go to the American Association of Christian Counselors and search your location. Many counselors are also willing to provide online support. https://connect.aacc.net/?search_type=distance

11. Guided Imagery/Visualizations - "Guided Meditation | Guided Imagery and Visualization | Health Journeys." www.healthjourneys.com
12. Healing Prayer - Approach your church about having them pray for your healing. You can also join HealingStrong™ during Prayer times. See https://healingstrong.org/refresh for times and zoom link.
13. Music - The saying goes "Stress is a killer, but music is a healer" (author unknown). Listening to uplifting or calming music helps soothe the soul, which has a cyclical effect reducing stress.
14. Gratitude - This is the practice of expressing gratitude daily. Some also recommend gratitude journaling.

Good, Better, Best Tips

Introduction for section on Good Better Best:

As each lesson concludes, we want to leave you with an idea(s) for how to implement a suggestion from the lesson in an incremental fashion that meets your needs and abilities. Each lesson will give you ideas that are "Good, Better, and Best".

Good Tips: A perfect way to get started implementing healthier healing options. This tip will be less involved from both a time, energy, effort and financial resources.

Better Tips: This tip will progress you further into implementing the lesson idea. More time and cost may be involved in this step.

Best Tips: When you are ready, this tip will give you ideas to help implement the lesson ideas in a more extensive fashion. This could mean significant investment of time, energy, effort, and financial resources.

LESSON 9:

Good: You are a Child of God! Be LESS critical of self and begin accepting His GRACE into your life. Practice forgiveness and compassion of self and others. Try to see yourself as Jesus sees you, not how the world sees you, or even how you see you.

Better: Identify the areas of stress in your life. Be intentional to make a plan to reduce the stress in your life.

Best: Take time and effort to work on inner healing. Connect with a ministry like https://www.rakministry.com or https://www.journeyu.org and set up a time to meet with their inner healing prayer team and begin to release emotions that have had a continuous impact on your overall well-being.

Discussion Questions/Action Steps:

1. Would anyone like to share which emotional area you struggle with the most?
   _____
   _____
   _____

2. In this lesson, did you learn any new ways to address emotional issues that you believe may help you?
   _____
   _____
   _____

3. Does anyone have a favorite affirmation that you use already?
   _____
   _____
   _____

4. Does anyone have any creative ways that you've found helpful in funding your healing protocol?
   _____
   _____
   _____

5. Has anyone used any of the strategies or emotional healing techniques we talked about today
   _____
   _____
   _____

CONNECT:

As a participant in a HealingStrong™ group, you have much to take advantage of in your healing journey. Our meetings are just a part of helping you on a consistent basis. Review these resources for things that can help Rebuild, Renew, and Refresh you all month long!

HealingStrong™ website: http://healingstrong.org
HealingStrong™ Facebook page: http://www.facebook.com/healingstrong/
HealingStrong™ Instagram page: https://www.instagram.com/healingstrongofficial/
HealingStrong™ I AM HealingStrong™ Podcast page: https://healingstrong.org/podcast
HealingStrong™ Start Here: https://healingstrong.org/start-here

Remember: "Fear is detrimental to healing, but affirmations based on God's Word help us replace it with courage and strength."

FIYAA AFFIRMATIONS

I will:

- **Forgive** myself and others.
- **Invite** God into all aspects of my life and healing.
- **Yield** to the needs of my body during this healing season.
- **Accept** my diagnosis and symptoms as temporary.
- **Abandon** negative expectations and think possibilities.

WWW.HEALINGSTRONG.ORG

Being a faith-based organization, we are not only passionate about your present healing journey, but also passionate about your eternal destiny as well. Of course, there will come an end to this life for all of us. We want to make sure that we have shared with you how to know that your eternal destiny is in heaven with our Creator, the One who formed you, loves you, and made a simple way for you to know for certain. If you are not a believer in Jesus Christ and would like to learn more about His saving grace, please see these resources: https://healingstrong.org/refresh

NOTES

Lesson 9 Additional Resources for Further Use

"The Cancer Personality: The Traits & How to Change Your Future". *Breast Cancer Conqueror.* 22 Feb 2022. Web. <https://breastcancerconqueror.com/the-cancer-personality/>.

Dr. Rutland, Mark. **Courage to be Healed: Finding Hope to Restore Your Soul.** Charisma House, 3 September 2019. Print.

Stockdale, Brenda. **You Can Beat the Odds: The Surprising Factors behind Chronic Illness and Cancer.** Sentient Publications. 1 Dec. 2009. Print.

God's love calms all my fears.

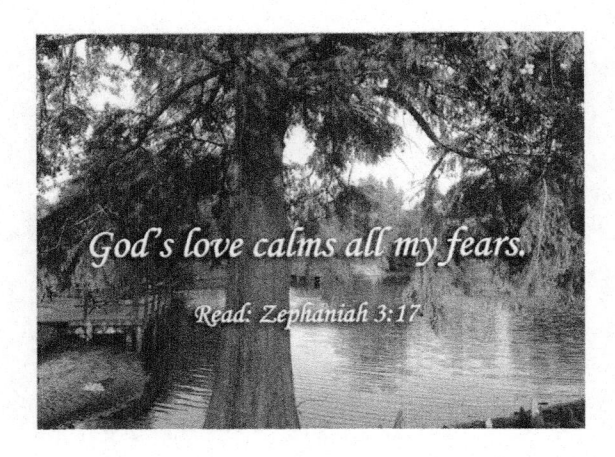

Read: Zephaniah 3:17

Dear Lord,

I am thankful You love me enough to continually grow me. I thank you that I am not yet who You have created me to be; but that by Your grace, I can become something greater!

Per Isaiah 43:18-19 (ESV) **"Remember not the former things, nor consider the things of old. Behold, I am doing a new thing, now it springs forth, do you not perceive it?"** Please help me to perceive the new life You would spring forth in me.

Finally, brothers and sisters, whatever is true, whatever is noble, whatever is right, whatever is pure, whatever is lovely, whatever is admirable - if anything is excellent or praiseworthy-think about such things. **- Philippians 4:8 NIV**

Thank you for the promises in Your word. Amen.

Soothing Soup

- 1 small sweet onion, chopped
- 3 cloves garlic, chopped
- 1 Tablespoon coconut oil
- 1 large sweet potato, peeled and chopped
- 2 organic carrots, scrubbed and medium diced
- 1 can 15 ounce organic white beans, drained & rinsed
- 2 cups cooked lentils
- 3 cups vegetable stock

Garnish
- 1 avocado, chopped
- ½ cup raw, chopped cashews

Sauté onion and garlic in coconut oil over low heat until translucent. Add in sweet potato and carrots. Stir for a couple of minutes to season root vegetables. Add stock and simmer for 15 minutes or until carrots and potato are tender. Add in spinach, beans and lentils and heat thoroughly.

Serve with chopped avocado and cashews sprinkled on top.

Lesson 10:
Exercise

> **NOTE:** The full Participant Guide is available for download at our Start Here Page https://healingstrong.org/start-here. Please also review our full disclaimer for HealingStrong™ at: https://healingstrong.org/start-here.

Lesson Objective & Key Concepts

Take Away/Objective:
The body is designed to move. Exercise aids the body in the detoxification process. It strengthens the overall condition of the body, boosts endorphins and serotonin, and makes your muscles stronger and more reactive. After all, if you don't USE it, you LOSE it!

Key Concepts:

- Embrace the importance of using movement to aid in healing.
- Exercise does not have to be rigorous or complicated.
- Rebounding combines exercise and detoxification.
- Proper walking is a good place to start exercising.
- Focus on injury prevention with strength conditioning.

DISCUSSION POINTS

***Note to the Reader:** Although lessons are geared towards healing from cancer, these lessons are educational in nature and offer information that will equip and empower you with health choices and action steps that you can take that may benefit your overall well-being. If you are on a healing protocol, whether preventative in nature, or treatment that is conventional, holistic or integrative, the principles taught in these lessons may be applied towards a supportive plan for many health challenges.

Why should we exercise, and how does it help your prognosis?

Exercise may protect against cancer and tumor development by serving to enhance energy balance, hormone metabolism, immune function, regulation of insulin production, and helping to move carcinogenic substances out of the body. It also reduces inflammation, which most experts agree is the cause of cancer and other chronic diseases.

Exercise must be included as part of a holistic healing regimen, not only to detoxify, but also to improve emotional health through boosting serotonin, our "happy hormone" levels in the brain.

You want to look for types of movement that focus on functional fitness. Functional fitness emphasizes whole body wellness through enhancing spinal health, biomechanical alignment, and increased range of motion. The basic aim is to move better in every possible way, resulting in overall resilience and injury resistance. Movement serves as an internal massage to stimulate every cell. This stimulation encourages detoxification, and enhances the ability of each cell to absorb oxygen and nutrients.

Preferred methods of movement address spinal mobility. The spinal cord is part of the central nervous system sending and receiving communication throughout the body. Good spinal health involves flexibility, and decompression of vertebrae promoting a healthy nervous system and circulation throughout the body. It can also aid in reduction of back pain and improve posture which improves breathing.

Rigorous exercise with muscle building is not recommended, since it could overtax the body by forcing it to rebuild large amounts of muscle tissue, while trying to heal from disease. This energy is needed to support the function of other organs and the immune system. This is especially true for those who are in active healing from cancer or other diseases.

Recommended exercises are:
- Brisk walking with or without light hand weights*
- Light, moderate distance running*
- Light to moderate hiking*
- Rebounding
- Swimming (preferably in a salt water pool to avoid the chemical chlorine)

- Dance or aerobics
- Light bicycling
- Mind-Body Movement

* If you have pain or discomfort with walking, moderate walking, or hiking, consider gait analysis to correct muscular imbalances. Some shoe stores can do this. There are many good online resources that address this as well including:

- https://www.youtube.com/watch?v=2BfbiyIKnK4
- https://www.corewalking.com/causes-and-treatment-for-hip-pain-when-walking/
- https://www.corewalking.com/walking-and-lower-back-pain-post2/

Create a Schedule

A common reason people do not exercise is time. Lengthy, lofty exercise goals can discourage anything from being accomplished. If this is YOU, then start small. Your goal should be to exercise 30-50 minutes daily, even if you have to break it up into 10 or 15 minute increments. There are several ways to do this.

- Develop an on the hour exercise plan by completing a 5 or 10 minute exercise on the hour for as many sessions as you set for yourself.
    - Setting an alarm on your phone is a helpful reminder. How about a 5 minute dance break? Or 5 minutes on your rebounder?
    - If you choose to move on the hour for just 5 minutes, five times a day, you would have already exercised 25 minutes!
- Talk with friends and family about how they incorporate movement into their lives.
- Consider a gym membership, a dance class, a tennis team, a fitness tracker bracelet, online accountability, or exercise videos. A good source for free videos can be found here: https://www.energyup.co.
- Ask yourself - What do you like to do? Would you rather move in a meditative, private way, or do you prefer to be with other people while you exercise? Doing what you enjoy will give you a good indicator that what you've chosen is a good fit for your needs at this time.
- Remember if you are in a healing season, strenuous exercise may not be the best choice. You want to feel energized rather than depleted by how you are moving!
- Create a checklist each day.
- Ask someone to be your accountability partner to encourage or exercise with you. Discovering fresh ways to move may also help with creating and maintaining your new habit.
- Outdoor exercise is highly recommended, if possible, for the fresh air and natural Vitamin D from the sun. Listen to healing scripture or uplifting music, or simply enjoy the silence or sounds of nature.

Overall, exercise is one more way you are empowering your body to heal itself the way God intended. You are strengthening your natural abilities towards healing while releasing toxins. Releasing those toxins improves your body's ability to repair.

Rebounding

You might wonder how jumping on a mini-trampoline could help with a diagnosis, but the science behind rebounding is both interesting and convincing. Rebounding is a fun, and HIGHLY effective form of exercise. You are essentially weightless at the top of each jump, allowing your cells to decompress. You land with twice the force of gravity on each bounce, which causes your cells to compress. This compression acts similarly to a sponge being squeezed out releasing cellular waste, while fresh nutrients and oxygen are pulled into each cell during decompression. Instead of lifting weight away FROM gravity to exercise the cells in a single muscle group, rebounding increases the weight OF gravity, thereby exercising ALL of your body's cells SIMULTANEOUSLY! In addition, this accelerated/decelerated bounce has MANY health benefits, including allowing the valves in your lymph system to open and close simultaneously, thus optimizing the flow of lymph fluid. Researchers at the University of Kentucky, in conjunction with NASA, concluded that "the magnitude of the biomechanical stimuli is greater with jumping on a trampoline than with running." (https://pubmed.ncbi.nlm.nih.gov/7429911/) More simply put, jumping on a rebounder flexes and massages every cell without added joint pressure and does it more effectively than more popular exercises. A simple "health-bounce" of a few inches up and down will increase circulation and flush your entire lymphatic system within a couple minutes.
Additional benefits of rebounding include:
- Increases cardiovascular fitness
- Greater balance and agility
- Improves circulation and blood pressure
- Reverses hardening of arteries
- Detoxifies the liver
- Improves digestion and elimination
- Lowers elevated cholesterol & triglyceride levels

There are several companies that make quality rebounders. Some are designed to function more smoothly, others to be easier on joints, while some are easier for travel and storage. Research different brands and types of rebounders before purchasing one. We suggest rebounding, not only for detoxification but also for a fun and unique way of exercise. (For more information, see http://www.anticancermom.com/detox-jump-around/).

Walking

If you are not already exercising, walking can be a good place to start. It doesn't require special equipment or athletic ability and offers great health benefits from joint lubrication, weight loss to improved mood, blood sugar control, improved lymph flow, and lowered blood pressure. Per an article in the Harvard Gazette (https://news.harvard.edu/gazette/story/2012/11/how-much-exercise-is-enough) adding 150 minutes of brisk walking to your routine each week can add 3.4 years to your lifespan. Unlike running, which is a high impact exercise, walking is gentle, and has a much lower potential for injury. Walking also prompts a chemical release of serotonin, the natural "feel good" chemical, while giving us an opportunity to nourish our mind and enjoy the quiet space to focus on positive, uplifting things.

Think about this while walking:

"Finally, brothers and sisters, whatever is true, whatever is noble, whatever is right, whatever is pure, whatever is lovely, whatever is admirable—if anything is excellent or praiseworthy—think about such things." Phil. 4:8 (NIV)

Turn walking time into a time of gratitude. Thank God for the good things in your life, even if all you can think of at the moment is the ability to put one foot in front of the other.

To take walking "a step" further, studies show that walking barefoot on the earth is of clinical significance. This is called: earthing. Walking barefoot has gone from being "a kooky counter-culture trend, to a scientifically researched practice with a number of remarkable health advantages, such as increasing antioxidants, reducing inflammation, and improving sleep." An article published in the Journal of Environmental Public Health states:

"Environmental medicine generally addresses environmental factors with a negative impact on human health. However, emerging scientific research has revealed a surprisingly positive and overlooked environmental factor on health: direct physical contact with the vast supply of electrons on the surface of the Earth. Modern lifestyle separates humans from such contact. The research suggests that this disconnect may be a major contributor to physiological dysfunction and un-wellness. Reconnection with the Earth's electrons has been found to promote intriguing physiological changes and subjective reports of well-being. Earthing (or grounding) refers to the discovery of benefits-including better sleep and reduced pain-from walking barefoot outside or sitting, working, or sleeping indoors connected to conductive systems that transfer the Earth's electrons from the ground into the body. This paper reviews the earthing research and the potential of earthing as a simple and easily accessed global modality of significant clinical importance."
(https://www.ncbi.nlm.nih.gov/pmc/articles/PMC3265077/)

Strength Conditioning Training and Weight Lifting

By sheer definition, strength conditioning is designed to enhance athletic performance. Building muscle, increasing strength, speed and agility are the primary objectives of strength conditioning. If you do incorporate strength conditioning as part of your routine, you will need to ensure that you are focused on injury prevention first, followed by performance enhancement. Using movement quality and mechanical efficiency to support weight training or a high intensity class can improve your outcome. It is always recommended to partner with a strength training coach to help you get started in this arena.

Important: Assess where you are at this moment. You may need to start with rebounding, walking, or mind-body movement before incorporating any focused strength conditioning. Creating a lifestyle of movement should be your first priority.

Mind-Body Movement

Mind-body movement combines mental focus with exercise, emphasizing breathing, muscular alignment, and purposeful action. It can help improve clarity of thought, ability to relax, and sleep quality. Mind-body movement also improves function of the nervous, hormonal, digestive, cardiovascular, pulmonary, and immune systems while boosting physical stamina and flexibility. Mind-body movement can help enhance awareness of the body and physical needs, growing an appreciation of the design of the body as you stretch and move.

Good, Better, Best Tips

Introduction for section on Good Better Best:

As each lesson concludes, we want to leave you with an idea(s) for how to implement a suggestion from the lesson in an incremental fashion that meets your needs and abilities. Each lesson will give you ideas that are "Good, Better, and Best".

Good Tips: A perfect way to get started implementing healthier healing options. This tip will be less involved from both a time, energy, effort and financial resources.

Better Tips: This tip will progress you further into implementing the lesson idea. More time and cost may be involved in this step.

Best Tips: When you are ready, this tip will give you ideas to help implement the lesson ideas in a more extensive fashion. This could mean significant investment of time, energy, effort, and financial resources.

LESSON 10:

Good: Make a 30+ min walk part of your daily schedule. Outside and barefoot when possible. Use the time to mentally offer up to God gratitude for your daily blessings or give thought to the things in life that bring you JOY. *Finally, brothers and sisters, whatever is true, whatever is noble, whatever is right, whatever is pure, whatever is lovely, whatever is admirable—if anything is excellent or praiseworthy—think about such things. Phillipians 4:8 NIV*

Better: Rebounding is the perfect option to increase your exercise level beyond a daily walk. If "jumping" is uncomfortable, use a gentle bounce. Set a timer and include 2-3 min of rebounding every hour, or 10-15 minutes a couple of times a day.

Best: Exercise to a good healthy sweat – increase your walking/bouncing to a more intensive jog or jump to really get your heart rate up and increase blood flow. Include a strength training exercise 3-4X a week. Explore different forms of movement and engage in those that give you joy and peace when moving!

Discussion Questions/Action Steps:

1. Assess your daily exercise level. Are you scheduling time to move on a daily basis?

   _____
   _____
   _____
   _____

2. If you are not getting enough exercise, what can you realistically add to your current activity level?

   _____
   _____
   _____
   _____

3. Do you enjoy movement more if you are socializing while exercising? Can you find someone to spend time with while moving? Perhaps at a class, or meeting together to walk in your neighborhood? Think about ways to enjoy adding more movement to your life!

   _____
   _____
   _____
   _____

4. What is your goal for this month? What are some obstacles? Tell someone in the group what you want to accomplish and how you plan to do it.

   _____
   _____
   _____
   _____

CONNECT:

As a participant in a HealingStrong™ group, you have much to take advantage of in your healing journey. Our meetings are just a part of helping you on a consistent basis. Review these resources for things that can help Rebuild, Renew, and Refresh you all month long!

HealingStrong™ website: http://healingstrong.org
HealingStrong™ Facebook page: http://www.facebook.com/healingstrong/
HealingStrong™ Instagram page: https://www.instagram.com/healingstrongofficial/
HealingStrong™ I AM HealingStrong™ Podcast page: https://healingstrong.org/podcast
HealingStrong™ Start Here: https://healingstrong.org/start-here

Remember: "Fear is detrimental to healing, but affirmations based on God's Word help us replace it with courage and strength."

FIYAA AFFIRMATIONS

I will:

- **Forgive** myself and others.
- **Invite** God into all aspects of my life and healing.
- **Yield** to the needs of my body during this healing season.
- **Accept** my diagnosis and symptoms as temporary.
- **Abandon** negative expectations and think possibilities.

WWW.HEALINGSTRONG.ORG

Being a faith-based organization, we are not only passionate about your present healing journey, but also passionate about your eternal destiny as well. Of course, there will come an end to this life for all of us. We want to make sure that we have shared with you how to know that your eternal destiny is in heaven with our Creator, the One who formed you, loves you, and made a simple way for you to know for certain. If you are not a believer in Jesus Christ and would like to learn more about His saving grace, please see these resources: https://healingstrong.org/refresh

NOTES

Lesson 10 Additional Resources for Further Use

#1 rebounder mini-trampolines by Needak Mfg. recommended by Dr. Morton Walker. (n.d.). 18 Dec. 2015. Web. <http://www.needak-rebounders.com/jumping-for-health.php>. (Note: HealingStrong™ does not necessarily recommend this rebounder as the number one; however, the website is a great resource on rebounding.)

Sileo, Dean. **Rebounding Demonstration** by *Sileo Wellness*. Film. <https://drive.google.com/file/d/1offzWrkURZ85t7AJFkRiW6tsOKcxDZy7/view>.

"The Benefits of Exercise during Cancer Treatment". *Cancer Exercise Training Institute*. 22 July 2022. Web. <https://www.thecancerspecialist.com/2022/07/27/exercise-during-cancer-treatment-2/>.

"The Benefits of Rebounding in the Prevention and Management of Lymphedema & improving Your Immune Resp". *Cancer Exercise Training Institute (CETI)*. 1 Aug 2019. Web. <https://www.thecancerspecialist.com/2019/08/01/the-benefits-of-rebounding-in-the-prevention-and-management-of-lymphedema/>.

"Physical Activity and Cancer". (n.d.). 18 Dec. 2015. Web. <http://www.cancer.gov/about-cancer/causes-prevention/risk/obesity/physical-activity-fact-sheet#q4>

"Why a Walking Workout is Good for Your Body". (n.d.). *Daily Mail*. 18 Dec. 2015. Web. <http://www.dailymail.co.uk/health/article-122898/Why-walking-workout-good-body.html#ixzz3udj8JvCD>.

> I sought God with all my heart... and found him.
>
> Read Deuteronomy 4:29

Raw Sweet Potato Brownies

- 1 large sweet potato, baked, cooled, peeled & mashed
- 1 cup raw pecans, finely chopped in food processor
- 1 cup raw cashews, finely chopped in food processor
- 1/3 cup raw cacao powder
- pinch Himalayan sea salt
- ¼ cup melted coconut oil
- ¼ cup maple syrup

Put all ingredients into a medium bowl and mix well. Pat firmly into a pan lightly greased with coconut oil. Refrigerate for at least 2 hours. Cut into small squares. Eat refrigerated squares within 3 days. Can be frozen for up to 1 month. let thaw 15 minutes before enjoying.

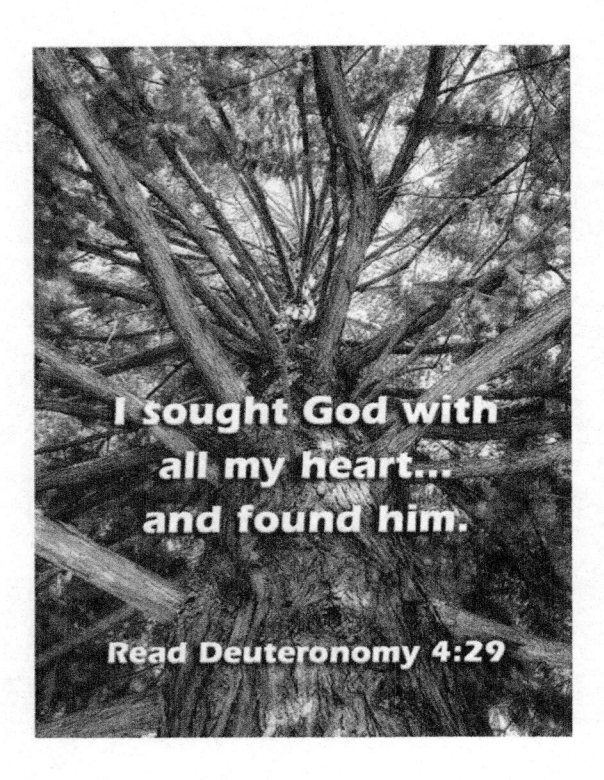

Dear Our Precious Lord,

Precious Lord and Savior, Jesus Christ – giver of eternal life,

Thank you for being with me on my journey ahead. Help me to travel down this foreign road. When I come to the wilderness, guide me. I trust You to keep me strong until the passage is finished.

For this reason I kneel before the Father, from whom His whole family in heaven and on earth derives its name. I pray that out of His glorious riches He may strengthen you with power through His Spirit in your inner being, so that Christ may dwell in your hearts through faith. And I pray that you, being rooted and established in love, may have power, together with all believers, to grasp how wide and long and high and deep is the love of Christ, and to know this love that surpasses knowledge – that you may be filled to the measure of all the fullness of God. Now to Him who is able to immeasurably more than all we ask or imagine, according to His power that is at work within us, to Him be glory in the Church and in Christ Jesus throughout all generation, forever and ever! Amen.
- Ephesians 3:14-21 NIV

Thank you for the promises in Your word. Amen.

Lesson 11:
Dental Toxins and Their Impact on Your Health

> **NOTE:** The full Participant Guide is available for download at our Start Here Page https://healingstrong.org/start-here. Please also review our full disclaimer for HealingStrong™ at: https://healingstrong.org/start-here.

LESSON OBJECTIVES & KEY CONCEPTS

Take Away Objective:
As much as we focus on detoxing and nutrition, dental clean-up is an important component, since one of the most contributing factors to ongoing health issues is right inside the mouth. We must recognize and address dental issues that have an impact on our body's ability to heal.

Key Concepts:

- Develop a daily dental routine that is the safest, least toxic way to achieve appropriate dental care. This should include reducing pathogens.

- Understand the importance of mercury-free dentistry, and address past dental procedures containing this toxin. Identify a biological and mercury free dentist, who can provide future dental education and care.

- Know the dangers of root canals.

- Identify natural remedies and nutrients to support heavy metal detoxification.

Discussion Points

***Note to the Reader: Although lessons are geared towards healing from cancer, these lessons are educational in nature and offer information that will equip and empower you with health choices and action steps that you can take that may benefit your overall well-being. If you are on a healing protocol, whether preventative in nature, or treatment that is conventional, holistic or integrative, the principles taught in these lessons may be applied towards a supportive plan for many health challenges.**

Dental Health

As you focus on your healing journey, it is important to remove the toxins from your body and maintain proper oral and dental health. The state of your mouth can have a profound impact on your ability to heal. Most of us have fillings, and many of us have had root canals done. It is important to understand the direct connection between your oral health and your overall health.

- Like many areas of the body, your mouth is full of bacteria. Normally the body's natural defenses plus routine oral health care, such as daily brushing and flossing, can keep bacteria under control. However, without proper oral hygiene, bacteria can reach levels that might lead to oral infections, such as tooth decay and gum disease. It is important to remove the toxins from your body and maintain proper dental health as part of your focused healing process.

- One simple way to instantly address dental pathogens and detox the mouth is to add oil pulling to your daily dental care regimen. Oil pulling is an ancient Ayurvedic dental technique, which draws out toxins and improves oral health by swishing oil (coconut, olive, or sesame), in the mouth on an empty stomach for around 20 minutes and then releasing it into a plastic cup that you can throw into the trash. To see how, watch Dr. Axe's video: https://www.youtube.com/watch?v=DtFzd3TBYil.

- It is important to floss every night. Dental tape removes more plaque; however, avoid teflon-coated floss. Most people do not floss deeply enough. The floss should go under the gum alongside each tooth. When brushing, use a soft brush and at a 45 degree angle toward the gum line. Use short, back and forth or circular strokes so the gums feel like they are getting a gentle massage.

- Fluoride is one of the most toxic elements, so use fluoride-free toothpaste.

- Drinking clean, fluoride-free water is critical. Obtain a good consumer brand water filtration system that removes fluoride from the water. An example is the Berkey Water filtration system. (Learn more about products we believe in and support the mission of HealingStrong™ at the bottom of this page: http://healingstrong.org/resources)

- If the gums bleed when brushing and flossing, that is a sign that the gums are infected with bacterial plaque and are inflamed as a result. This plaque must be removed for the gums to heal, even if it causes bleeding.

- If plaque is not removed daily, minerals from saliva are deposited into it, and it hardens into calculus or tartar. This usually cannot be removed by brushing and flossing and requires professional cleaning at a dental office. If left untreated, the bacteria will infect and destroy the bone that holds the teeth into the jaw. This is gum disease and it is how teeth are lost.

Cavities

- The most common filling material used for more than 150 years has been "silver" amalgam fillings. They are called silver fillings even though they contain more mercury than silver, as well as various other metals.
- Mercury is the most toxic, naturally occurring metal and is used in silver amalgam fillings consisting of 55% of the material base. See: https://iaomt.org/resources/dental-mercury-facts/dental-mercury-amalgam-side-effects/. The mercury vapor that is emitted when one chews, eats, drinks hot beverages, or brushes the teeth is more dangerous than the mercury itself. A very helpful demonstration of the release of mercury vapor during chewing or brushing can be seen here: SMOKING TEETH - https://www.youtube.com/watch?v=9ylnQ-T7oiA.
- Safely removing the mercury is an important consideration to the healing process. In order to understand the impact mercury has on the body, it is important to examine research associated with mercury toxicity. Mercury was first introduced as a filling by the English chemist, Bell, in 1819 (per http://www.toothbythelake.net/wellness-center/amalgam-fillings/a-brief-history-of-amalgams/). Despite harmful effects so widely reported, use has continued to this day.
- The American Dental Association (ADA) is a pro-amalgam faction, and in spite of research reports of harmful effects, it continued to sit in silence when a 2013 United Nations treaty signed by over ninety countries aimed at reducing global mercury usage, including reducing dental mercury. See: https://en.wikipedia.org/wiki/Minamata_Convention_on_Mercury. Research shows more than 67 million Americans aged two years and older exceed the intake of mercury vapor considered "safe" by the US Environmental Protection Agency due to the presence of dental amalgam fillings in their mouth. See: https://iaomt.org/resources/dental-mercury-facts/dental-amalgam-safety-myth-truth/.

Health Problems Associated With Mercury

Mercury is known to be the most toxic, naturally-occurring metal on the planet. Mercury fillings have been known to cause health issues in the nerves, at the cellular level (cytotoxic), and broader immune level (immunotoxic) such as:

- Heart disease
- Fatigue
- Headaches
- Respiratory problems
- Dermatological conditions
- Neurological problems, including depression, memory loss, anxiety, and fine tremors

See: https://iaomt.org/resources/dental-mercury-facts/mercury-poisoning-symptoms-dental-amalgam/).

Since this poison damages the immune system, if you are on a healing journey, removal of the mercury fillings is an important consideration. If you cannot remove the fillings, then it is important to look at nutrition and supplements that help detoxify the body of heavy metals. Dr. Joseph Mercola and Chris Slade provide viewers a great overview of three pillars to heavy metal detoxification: http://realhealthcareclinic.com/2016/10/the-three-pillars-of-heavy-metal-detoxification/

Removal of mercury from your teeth can be quite costly in most countries. There are very reputable clinics in the United States and other countries that the larger cancer hospitals such as Hope 4 Cancer or Gerson Clinic encourage their patients to see. Finding the right practitioner is important and praying through how to use the funds you have is another consideration. Do lots of research and interview other patients who have done it. Your HealingStrong™ group is a great place to start. Remember, HealingStrong™ doesn't believe you have to mortgage your house or go bankrupt in order to heal. There are ways to daily detox that can support your healing and cost much less than a complete dental overhaul.

The Fluoride Myth

In the following 20 minute video, attorney Michael Connett summarizes FACTS about fluoride issues. https://www.youtube.com/watch?v=GX0s-4AyWfI

In summary, most advanced countries do not fluoridate their water...and compared to non-fluoridated water, there is not a significant decline in tooth decay. This report based on the World Health Organization data indicates there is no discernible difference between countries that fluoridate and those that don't - https://fluoridealert.org/studies/caries01/. Fluoride toxicity studies indicate that fluoride contributes to many health issues that affect the bone, thyroid gland, pineal gland, and pancreas. It especially affects those who are immunocompromised by cancer and other diseases. Fluoridation is not a natural process. Studies have shown that fluoride is linked to the following health problems per https://fluoridealert.org/issues/health/:

- Arthritis
- Bone fractures
- Brain effects
- IQ loss
- Cancer
- Cardiovascular disease
- Diabetes
- Endocrine disruption
- Gastrointestinal effects
- Kidney disease
- Male fertility
- Pineal gland
- Thyroid disease

Be Informed. Know the Alternatives.

- The International Academy of Oral Medicine and Toxicology (http://iaomt.org/) offers advice to patients and dentists on mercury free dentistry, in addition to providing a list of dentists who are accredited as mercury free. The website includes information about safe materials usage, as well as information for patients, regarding the process of removing amalgam fillings.
- There are many alternatives to amalgam that can be used for restoration of decay and diseased teeth. When choosing a dentist, it is important to find out what kind of mercury-free restorations are used in their practice. Some safe examples may include composites or ceramics.
- You may also want to request a dental materials reactivity test or bioenergetic dental testing to help determine the compatibility of various options and how they react with your immune system. When you employ a biocompatible dentist, he/she can help you find a testing site to determine the best materials that are biocompatible with your immune system. This is a safe and relatively inexpensive test that will help you and your dentist make the best choice for restorative materials.

Detoxing Mercury

- Mercury exits through the liver, kidney, skin, and exhaled air. It is important when you detox to work with a knowledgeable health professional. Consider testing for adequate levels of nutrients such as vitamin C, selenium, glutathione, and zinc.
- Intestinal binders, free of impurities, can be helpful. Examples are bentonite clay, activated charcoal, and zeolite. Greens, especially cilantro and chlorella, are advantageous. Juicing these greens or taking in supplement form helps to pull mercury out of the body.

Root Canal

- Root Canal is a procedure performed when a tooth becomes extremely infected in an attempt to save the badly decayed tooth. The procedure removes the nerve and pulp in the tooth and replaces it with permanent dental material. Once the procedure is complete, your tooth is dead.
- It is important to note that our teeth are part of the intricate lymph and blood system. Teeth are fed from their roots by the dentinal lymph system. The tooth structure is composed of small microscopic tubules, leading from the pulp inside the tooth to the outside of the tooth.
- When the pulp is removed, circulation to the tooth is cut. This allows anaerobic bacteria (bacteria that grow in the absence of oxygen) to proliferate inside the tubules of the teeth. This can produce toxins that can spread throughout the body, which can stress the immune system.
- The alternative to root canal treatment is to remove the tooth. For more information on root canals connection to cancer: https://thetruthaboutcancer.com/root-canals-cause-cancer/

Good, Better, Best Tips

Introduction for section on Good Better Best:
As each lesson concludes, we want to leave you with an idea(s) for how to implement a suggestion from the lesson in an incremental fashion that meets your needs and abilities. Each lesson will give you ideas that are "Good, Better, and Best".

Good Tips: A perfect way to get started implementing healthier healing options. This tip will be less involved from both a time, energy, effort and financial resources.

Better Tips: This tip will progress you further into implementing the lesson idea. More time and cost may be involved in this step.

Best Tips: When you are ready, this tip will give you ideas to help implement the lesson ideas in a more extensive fashion. This could mean significant investment of time, energy, effort, and financial resources.

LESSON 11:

Dr. Teresa Scott, Biological Dentist and speaker for HealingStrong encourages us to take time to learn how your dental health impacts your overall well-being. These good, better, best tips are written with the help of Dr. Scott.

Good Tips: Switch to a toothpaste that is free of the toxins often found in most commercial toothpastes or make your own. A simple paste can be made using equal parts of coconut oil and an aluminum free baking soda with a few drops of essential oil for flavor/antibacterial nature (i.e. grapefruit, peppermint, tea tree, orange, lemongrass, eucalyptus) Optional ingredients might include activated charcoal for whitening and natural clay or sea salt for remineralization. Stevia can be added as a sweetener. Many recipes can be found online. Adjust the ingredients/amounts to suit your preference.

Better Tips: Find a biological dentist to support you in all your cleaning and other dental support needs. Do your due diligence. You may have to visit several to find a good match for your needs.

Best Tips: Have your root canal and amalgam filled teeth evaluated by a certified biological dentist to determine if they are causing a burden to your body. If they are, especially root canaled teeth, work with a functional medicine doctor AND a biological dentist to prepare your body and remove and replace the problem fillings or teeth with more biocompatible options. Also, have your entire oral systemic system evaluated for oral contributions to systemic health issues by working with a functional medicine doctor and an airway centered biological dentist who understand the oral/systemic health connection to address.

Discussion Questions/Action Steps:

1. Have you considered how your dental health relates to your overall health? What surprises you? Is there anything you need to further research?

   _____
   _____
   _____
   _____
   _____
   _____
   _____

2. How can you clean up your daily dental care regimen? Maybe flossing or changing to a fluoride- free toothpaste is a starting point.

   _____
   _____
   _____
   _____
   _____
   _____
   _____

3. What is your goal for this month? What are some obstacles? Tell someone in the group what you want to accomplish and how you plan to do it.

   _____
   _____
   _____
   _____
   _____
   _____

CONNECT:

As a participant in a HealingStrong™ group, you have much to take advantage of in your healing journey. Our meetings are just a part of helping you on a consistent basis. Review these resources for things that can help Rebuild, Renew, and Refresh you all month long!

HealingStrong™ website: http://healingstrong.org
HealingStrong™ Facebook page: http://www.facebook.com/healingstrong/
HealingStrong™ Instagram page: https://www.instagram.com/healingstrongofficial/
HealingStrong™ I AM HealingStrong™ Podcast page: https://healingstrong.org/podcast
HealingStrong™ Start Here: https://healingstrong.org/start-here

Remember: "Fear is detrimental to healing, but affirmations based on God's Word help us replace it with courage and strength."

FIYAA AFFIRMATIONS

I will:

- **Forgive** myself and others.
- **Invite** God into all aspects of my life and healing.
- **Yield** to the needs of my body during this healing season.
- **Accept** my diagnosis and symptoms as temporary.
- **Abandon** negative expectations and think possibilities.

WWW.HEALINGSTRONG.ORG

Being a faith-based organization, we are not only passionate about your present healing journey, but also passionate about your eternal destiny as well. Of course, there will come an end to this life for all of us. We want to make sure that we have shared with you how to know that your eternal destiny is in heaven with our Creator, the One who formed you, loves you, and made a simple way for you to know for certain. If you are not a believer in Jesus Christ and would like to learn more about His saving grace, please see these resources: https://healingstrong.org/refresh

NOTES

Lesson 11 Additional Resources for Further Use

"Dr. Tom McGuire's Mercury Safe Dentist Internet Directory." *Dr. Tom McGuire*. Web. <https://mercurysafedentists.net/>.

"How to Rid Your Body of Heavy Metals: A 3-Step Detoxification Plan - Dr. Mark Hyman." *Dr Mark Hyman*. 19 May 2010. Web. <http://drhyman.com/blog/2010/05/19/how-to-rid-your-body-of-mercury-and-other-heavy-metals-a-3-step-plan-to-recover-your-health/>.

"IAOMT MERCURY FILLINGS." IAOMT - International Academy of Oral Medicine and Toxicology. YouTube. 17 Sep. 2014. Film. <https://www.youtube.com/watch?v=i17bb21Cy50>.

"Mercury Infographic - Top 5 Facts on Mercury". *BioDental Healing*. 27 Jan 2016. Web. <https://www.biodentalhealing.com/blog/mercury-infographic-dr-villarreal/>.

"Meridian Tooth Chart." *Dr Elmira Gadol DMD Holistic Dentist*. 6 Mar. 2021. Web. <http://drgadol.com/meridian-tooth-chart/>.

"Mike Godfrey, MD Reviews the Adverse Effects of Mercury Fillings IAOMT L.V. 2007." IAOMT - International Academy of Oral Medicine and Toxicology. YouTube. 20 Aug. 2011. Web. <https://www.youtube.com/watch?v=lncLCWhm7o0>.

Monro-Hall, BDS, Dr. Graeme, and Dr Lilian Munro-Hall. **Toxic Dentistry Exposed: The Link Between Dentistry and Chronic Disease. 2nd ed.** Dr. Graeme Monro-Hall, BDS, 2009. Print.

"Search for IAOMT Member Dentists / Physicians - IAOMT." IAOMT - International Academy of Oral Medicine and Toxicology. Web. <https://iaomt.org/for-patients/search/>.

"Surprising Cancer Prevention Steps You've Never Thought Of!" *iHealthTube.com*. YouTube. 9 Jun. 2014. Web. <https://www.youtube.com/watch?v=PyBDMFuVaEw>.

"The Hidden Cause of Cavities and Tooth Decay." *Jing Soda®* YouTube. 18 Aug. 2015. Web. <https://www.youtube.com/watch?t=10&v=JD1MNupltio>.

Ziff, Sam, and Michael F. Ziff. **Dentistry without Mercury. Rev. & Expanded 1997 ed.** Orlando, Fla.: Bio-Probe, 1997. Print.

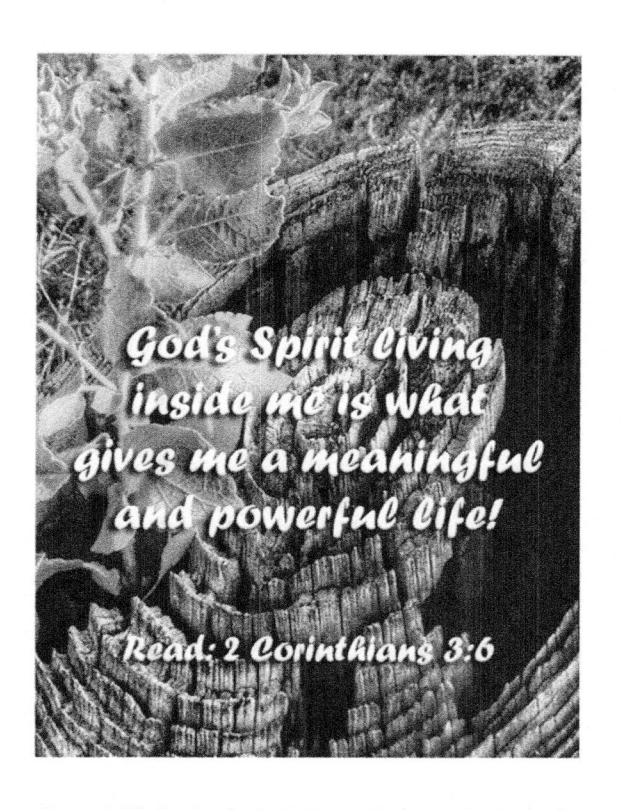

> God's Spirit living inside me is what gives me a meaningful and powerful life!
>
> Read: 2 Corinthians 3:6

Smoothie

- 1 avocado
- 1 handful spinach
- ¼ teaspoon ground turmeric
- 1 can coconut milk
- 1 cup coconut water
- ½ cup almonds, soaked overnight
- 2 Tablespoons chia seeds
- 2 Tablespoons maple syrup - or to taste
- 1 Tablespoon raw cacao powder

Blend all ingredients together until smooth.

Dear God,

Help me to bless Your name in good times and in bad. When I feel overwhelmed, be my strength. Through Jesus Christ our Lord. Amen.

**Bless the Lord, O my soul;
And all that is within me,
bless His holy name!**

**Bless the Lord, O my soul,
And forget not all His benefits:
Who forgives all your iniquity,
Who heals all your diseases,
Who redeems your life from the pit,
Who crowns you
with steadfast love and mercy.** - Psalm 103:1-4 ESV

Thank you for the promises in Your word. Amen.

Lesson 12:
Sleep, Meditation, and Breathing

> **NOTE:** The full Participant Guide is available for download at our Start Here Page https://healingstrong.org/start-here. Please also review our full disclaimer for HealingStrong™ at: https://healingstrong.org/start-here.

LESSON OBJECTIVE & KEY CONCEPTS

Take Away/Objectives:

Sleep is important and can't be ignored to heal the body and mind. Biblical meditation and breathing are daily practices that can be used to calm and cleanse the body and mind from the stresses of daily living while renewing the spirit.

Key Concepts:

- Sleep quality and quantity must be addressed in one's healing journey.
- Restful sleep plays an important role in aiding the immune system.
- There are techniques and strategies we can use to get better sleep.
- Meditating on God's word helps to renew the mind, calm the body, and restore the spirit by learning to listen to God and meditate on His Word.
- Taking time in meditation is an important habit to achieve and maintain healing.
- Proper breathing can calm and heal the nervous system. It is often a habit adults need to relearn.

DISCUSSION POINTS

***Note to the Reader:** Although lessons are geared towards healing from cancer, these lessons are educational in nature and offer information that will equip and empower you with health choices and action steps that you can take that may benefit your overall well-being. If you are on a healing protocol, whether preventative in nature, or treatment that is conventional, holistic or integrative, the principles taught in these lessons may be applied towards a supportive plan for many health challenges.

Sleep
- The minute your body slips into restful sleep, it begins to repair itself. There are five sleep cycles, each with unique functions, that prepare the body to live in health. See: https://www.psychologytoday.com/us/blog/between-you-and-me/201307/your-sleep-cycle-revealed.
- Achieving deep, restful sleep is the best way to ensure we get all of the healing benefits that come from each phase of sleep. To do this, sleep experts recommend seven to nine hours of sleep for adults and even more for children. See: https://www.sleephealthjournal.org/article/S2352-7218%2815%2900015-7/fulltext.

How Sleep Affects Cancer and Healing
- Two key hormones that work to boost our immune systems are produced during sleep. The first, cortisol, is a naturally occurring hormone that is most well-known for its role during times of stress, but it is also used to regulate our immune system and the production of natural killer cells during sleep, optimizing our natural ability to heal. Sleeping properly allows our natural cortisol cycle to work when it's supposed to.
- The other key hormone impacted by sleep is melatonin. Melatonin may have antioxidant properties that prevent damage to our healthy cells that could mutate to cause cancer. See: https://www.intechopen.com/chapters/62672. Melatonin also reduces levels of estrogen. Increased estrogen has been shown to result in higher incidence of breast cancer. See: https://calmerme.com/melatonin-anti-estrogenic/.
- Our cognitive ability to manage stress also works optimally when we get an adequate amount of sleep which benefits the whole body and mind.
- Maintaining healthy levels of the "stress hormones" cortisol and adrenaline are affected by the amount of sleep we get. When these hormones are out of whack, it can lead to increased inflammation which creates an environment for cancer cells to increase in number.

Tips for Better Healing Sleep
If you're finding yourself here in your own healing journey, whether from cancer or another disease, it is crucial that you make a strategic sleep schedule a priority. Here are some ways to help optimize your sleep.

- Ditch the night shift: Several studies linking night shift workers to increased cancer probabilities. One such study is https://www.huffpost.com/entry/stress-sleep-cancer_b_5063797. If it's absolutely necessary to work at night, get on a consistent sleeping schedule during the day.
- The human adult needs seven to nine hours of deep, uninterrupted sleep. Keep it predictable so your body is trained to sleep during a certain time.
- Invest in blackout curtains, if there is a lot of artificial light coming through your windows.
- Change your sheets every two weeks and make sure they are cool and comfortable. Consider the quality of your sheets. You may want organic cotton or organic bamboo to avoid absorbing chemicals from synthetic fabrics while you are sleeping.
- Make sure to eliminate lights from technology, alarm clocks, and other sources before sleep. Go ahead and turn off the technology, including cell phones, about an hour before bedtime to ensure that the light doesn't interfere with your natural wake/sleep cycle.
- If you need to use an alarm clock, consider buying a sunrise alarm clock.
- Turn off the wi-fi. You can set it on a timer!
- Make sure you are not sleeping close to an electrical "smart meter" by your house.
- Keep your room from 60-70 degrees. Studies show people sleep better in cooler air. See: https://www.sleepfoundation.org/bedroom-environment/best-temperature-for-sleep.
- Develop a routine before bed that helps you relax. This consistency helps cue the body that it is time to sleep. Sip chamomile tea, mentally make a gratitude list or take deep breaths to end the day on a calm, peaceful note to welcome sleep.
- Use essential oil in a diffuser or on your sheets. Lavender, ylang ylang, and others can be soothing. Add 10 to 20 drops of essential oil to two cups of distilled water for a quick linen spray.
- Use an earthing mat. See: https://www.healthline.com/health/under-review-grounding-mats#does-it-matter.
- Limit or prohibit caffeine use after 12pm.
- Use a sound conditioner or white noise machine.
- Certain supplements such as magnesium can help with better sleep.

Breathing and Meditation

HealingStrong™ pairs these two practices together along with sleep because meditation and breathing can actually help you achieve better sleep and relaxation.

Breathing

For optimal oxygen intake you need to learn how to breathe from your belly. To practice this in your chair put one hand on your belly below your navel and the rest the other on your chest. As you breathe in you should feel your belly rise not your chest. Practice breathing techniques at home.

Let's practice. Breathe in deeply through your nose for three seconds, hold for four seconds, then exhale for five seconds through your mouth. Repeat two to three times.

This is how we should aim to breathe every day, especially in times of stress or when trying to fall asleep. Consider choosing a trigger for remembering when to do this. Maybe it is when you have to stop for a stoplight when driving. Or maybe the trigger could be everytime you go to the restroom. It would be especially good to do this deep breathing outside in fresh air!

Meditating on God's Word

Meditation by definition is: "contemplation; devout preoccupation; devotions, prayer." The difference between Eastern Meditation and Discipline of Biblical Meditation: Eastern or New Age meditation is an effort to empty the mind in detachment, while the discipline of Biblical meditation, at its core, is a way of simplicity, silence, and stillness to hear God. It is a way to calm the mind and therefore the body, as we move towards greater attachment and connection with Him.

Meditation is an ancient spiritual practice in the Bible. You can find several verses that highlight the importance of meditation in His word at this link: http://bible.knowing-jesus.com/topics/Meditation. Here are a few verses:

> *How blessed is the man who does not walk in the counsel of the wicked, Nor stand in the path of sinners, Nor sit in the seat of scoffers! But his delight is in the law of the LORD, And in His law he meditates day and night. – Psalm 1:1-2 (KJV)*

> *Let the words of my mouth, and the meditation of my heart, be acceptable in thy sight, O LORD, my strength, and my redeemer. – Psalm 19:14 (KJV)*

We need to relax and quiet our minds on a daily basis. It is a nourishing part of the healing process allowing us to hear from God and our bodies. Meditation can be a big help as you learn to do this. Not only will this break the mental cycle of stress responses and feelings of frantic busy-ness, it can slow your heart beat and begin to normalize your blood pressure.

Tuning into the needs of your body can give confidence as you begin to trust your ability to heal. Hearing the whispers of the Holy Spirit can renew body and soul as God breathes new life into you during quiet times. It isn't difficult. Here's how to get started:

1. Find a comfortable position in a quiet place. Relax your body.
2. Let go of all thoughts (both good and bad), images, and other distractions. Just focus on your breath going in and out of your belly. Breathe in and out slowly for one to two minutes. It can be calming to place one hand on your heart and another on your abdomen just below your navel. Don't forget that this is a skill. It may take time to feel comfortable doing it.

3. Pick a word, prayer, or small verse of scripture to repeat slowly in your mind. For example, *"Come to me, all you who are weary and burdened, and I will give you rest." Matthew 11:28 (NASB)*. Also, *"Jesus is the same yesterday and today and forever." Hebrews 13:8 (NASB)*. A great set of verses to choose from are God's promises in the Bible. Here is one example set: https://www.compassionuk.org/blogs/gods-promises/.
4. Do this for a short amount of time, setting the stage for your meditation with your word, verse, or prayer. Work your way up to 10 to 20 minutes or longer.
5. After you have begun your time of meditation with your word, or verse, allow your thoughts to go where they will, trusting that God is directing you. You may find yourself becoming more aware of a physical or emotional issue affecting your healing, or feeling encouraged in a specific way as your time becomes more intimate with God. Let Him speak to you while you rest in His love for you.
6. Don't forget that this is a skill. It may take time to feel comfortable doing it.

Here are some ideas to meditate on God throughout the day:
- Upon waking, start with gratitude by thanking God for another day of life and for what the day will bring.
- Repeat the chosen word, prayer or small verse from your meditation session to reflect upon when you do the breathing exercise discussed above.
- Before you eat, thank God for the food. When you take your supplements, pray to God to bless their healthful benefits.
- Listen to worship music while doing chores, driving, or whenever you can.
- Put post-it notes around the house and/or work with scriptures that are important to you.
- See God in the little miracles, e.g. an insect hard at work on a plant, the mountains, a storm, conversations with others, a small child and their curiosity and zest for life. His handprints are on everything!
- Turn problems into praise as if they are already taken care of, because in the spiritual realm, they are. We are reminded of what *faith is - "Now faith is confidence in what we hope for and assurance about what we do not see." Hebrew 11:1 (NIV)*
- Set hourly reminders to take a quick break from whatever you are doing to stop and pray. This is especially helpful when you're feeling overwhelmed or fearful. It forces you to stop trying to do things in your own strength, and to surrender every hour to the Lord.
- When you lay down to sleep, review the blessings of the day and praise God for them.
- You can find 25 other ways to meditate on God throughout the day here - https://proverbs31mentor.com/25-ways-to-meditate-on-gods-word-throughout-the-day/.

Actual Practice for Visualization and Meditating on God

Tips for letting negative thoughts go so that your time does not become anxious:

- Imagine wrapping up your negative thoughts and letting Jesus take them from you.
- You can imagine worrisome thoughts and disease being blown away with each exhale while each inhale brings in the breath of life from God and His healing power.
- If you continue to have negative or intrusive thoughts, acknowledge them, mentally giving God permission to carry those difficulties for you, and re-focusing on His love for you and the goodness of the way He is healing your life and body.
- Take time to experiment with imagery and words that work for you, making space for Him to fill you with His peace and communion. It'll get easier as you practice!

An excellent resource that is inexpensive to download is Heaven's Health Food by Dr. Larry Hutton. On the CD or downloadable MP3 file, Dr. Hutton quotes Healing Scriptures from many translations in a unique way that will truly make God's Word come alive to you. It is an amazing resource to hear God's promises about healing over and over in various translations of the Bible. https://larryhutton.netviewshop.com/shopDetail/HHF1MP3

Based on Mark Virkler's book "4 Keys to Hearing God's Voice" is a free MP3 "A Stroll Along the Sea of Galilee" that you can play during your morning devotional time. It paints a scene of you and Jesus walking together along the Sea of Galilee then leads you into questions you could ask Him. It then guides you into how to hear the answers based on the four keys in Mark Virkler's book. You can access it at https://go.cwgministries.org/galilee-cwg.

Here is a free download of the Psalms being read with a recording of mountain streams in the background: https://mailchi.mp/healingstrong/39f58txjmq.

Good, Better, Best Tips

Introduction for section on Good Better Best:

As each lesson concludes, we want to leave you with an idea(s) for how to implement a suggestion from the lesson in an incremental fashion that meets your needs and abilities. Each lesson will give you ideas that are "Good, Better, and Best".

Good Tips: A perfect way to get started implementing healthier healing options. This tip will be less involved from both a time, energy, effort and financial resources.

Better Tips: This tip will progress you further into implementing the lesson idea. More time and cost may be involved in this step.

Best Tips: When you are ready, this tip will give you ideas to help implement the lesson ideas in a more extensive fashion. This could mean significant investment of time, energy, effort, and financial resources.

LESSON 12:

Here are tips to help you sleep better. *When you lie down, you will not be afraid, when you lie down, your sleep will be sweet. – Proverbs 3:24 NIV*

Good: Take the first step by creating a good sleep environment. Declutter your room. Make sure you have adequate bedding that is clean and not cluttered. Eat a diet that is healthy and remove the caffeine and other stimulants that may be keeping you awake at night.

Better: Put your wi-fi on a timer. Remove the television from your bedroom. Use blackout curtains and keep technology in another room.

Best: Use an earthing mat on your bed. See https://healthline.com/health/under-review-grounding-mats#does-it-matter

Discussion Questions/Action Steps:

1. By a show of hands, how many of you are getting seven to nine hours of sleep each night? What one or two things can you all do to improve your sleep tonight?

   _____
   _____
   _____
   _____
   _____

2. Do you have a daily quiet time and could you incorporate meditating on God's Word for healing?

   _____
   _____
   _____
   _____
   _____

3. Does anyone have any favorite scripture you prefer to meditate on for healing?

   _____
   _____
   _____
   _____
   _____

4. How do you tune in to God throughout the day?

   _____
   _____
   _____
   _____

CONNECT:

As a participant in a HealingStrong™ group, you have much to take advantage of in your healing journey. Our meetings are just a part of helping you on a consistent basis. Review these resources for things that can help Rebuild, Renew, and Refresh you all month long!

HealingStrong™ website: http://healingstrong.org
HealingStrong™ Facebook page: http://www.facebook.com/healingstrong/
HealingStrong™ Instagram page: https://www.instagram.com/healingstrongofficial/
HealingStrong™ I AM HealingStrong™ Podcast page: https://healingstrong.org/podcast
HealingStrong™ Start Here: https://healingstrong.org/start-here

Remember: "Fear is detrimental to healing, but affirmations based on God's Word help us replace it with courage and strength."

FIYAA AFFIRMATIONS

I will:

- **Forgive** myself and others.
- **Invite** God into all aspects of my life and healing.
- **Yield** to the needs of my body during this healing season.
- **Accept** my diagnosis and symptoms as temporary.
- **Abandon** negative expectations and think possibilities.

WWW.HEALINGSTRONG.ORG

Being a faith-based organization, we are not only passionate about your present healing journey, but also passionate about your eternal destiny as well. Of course, there will come an end to this life for all of us. We want to make sure that we have shared with you how to know that your eternal destiny is in heaven with our Creator, the One who formed you, loves you, and made a simple way for you to know for certain. If you are not a believer in Jesus Christ and would like to learn more about His saving grace, please see these resources: https://healingstrong.org/refresh

NOTES

Lesson 12 Additional Resources for Further Use

"18 Amazing Benefits of Chamomile Tea for Your Health." *Natural Remedy Ideas.* Web. <https://naturalremedyideas.com/chamomile-tea-benefits/>.

Bellew, Joni RN. **Nurse, Nurse, I'm Worse! Can You Help Me Sleep?**. Clovercroft Publishing. 2017 Print.

Bible Meditations: *Meditations on the Mount.* YouTube, n.d. Web. <https://www.youtube.com/channel/UCM94lE_vkmyur15J-Dk7Cwg/videos>.

Foster, Richard J. **Celebration of Discipline.** New York: Hodder & Stoughton, 1989. Print.

"HealingStrong Webinar: When you lie down, your sleep will be sweet". *HealingStrong™*. 27 Sep 2021. Web. <https://vimeo.com/712926836>.

"How to Use Melatonin 3mg tablet." *Web MD: Melatonin Use and Dosage.* Web. <http://www.webmd.com/drugs/drug-29-melatonin+oral.aspx>.

Letting Go of Anxiety and Fear - Christian Meditation - Meditations on the Mount. *Meditations on the Mount.* YouTube. 23 Dec. 2013. Web. <https://www.youtube.com/watch?v=qHYWMrH16Tk>.

"Sleep Products I Recommend." *Chris Wark, Chris Beat Cancer.* Web. <https://www.chrisbeatcancer.com/sleep-products-i-recommend/>.

The Christian Meditator YouTube Channel. *The Christian Meditator.* YouTube, n.d. Web. <https://www.youtube.com/c/Thechristianmeditator>.

"What is Meditation?." The World Community for Christian Meditation. Web. <http://wccm.org/content/what-meditation>.

> Jesus is my truth and way to an abundant Life & heaven.
>
> Read: John 14:6

Chocolate Protein Power Drink

- 1 cup organic old fashioned oats (variation: use quinoa flakes)
- 24 ounces - organic coconut water
- 2 heaping Tablespoons – Almond butter
- 1/8-1/4 cup (depending on your desired sweetness) – organic maple syrup
- 1 Tablespoon chia and/or hemp seeds
- 2 teaspoon organic raw cacao powder
- 1/4 cup dried mulberries
- 1/2 cup organic black beans (drained)
- 1 Tablespoon Bee Pollen
- Ice cubes
- Put all ingredients in your power blender (ie: Vitamix) and blend.

*(Note: Can also add cinnamon, or substitute blueberries, etc. **Variation:** To make this into a more hearty pudding or thicker shake, add avocado and chia seeds)*

Cream topping for the thicker variation:
Refrigerate overnight - can of organic coconut milk
Drain the clear liquid off the creamy mixture
In a bowl, mix the creamed coconut mixture with orange zest and 1-2 T maple syrup, with a dash of vanilla.

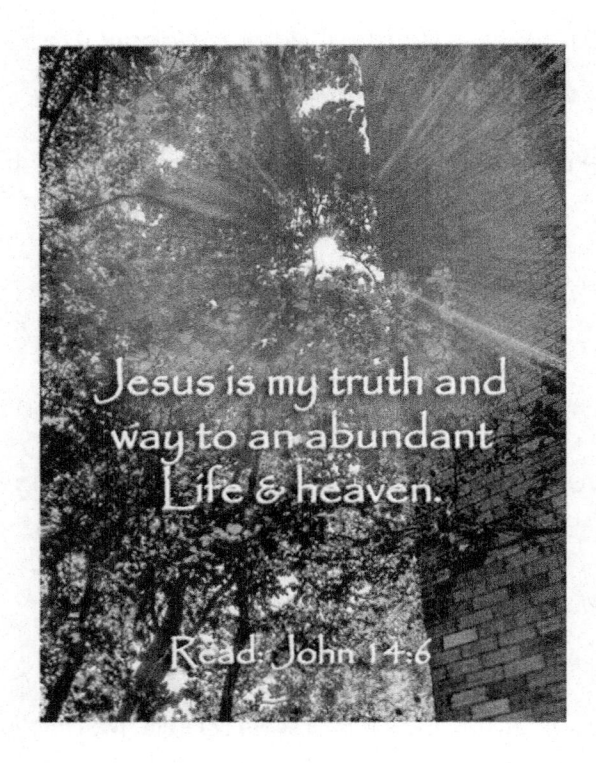

Your word says:

Now faith is confidence of what we hope for assurance about what we do not see. - Hebrews 11:1 NIV

Dear God,

You are our best compassion and the source of every comfort. Touch me with Your unfailing love and grace. You are close to those going through trials. See my struggles and respond when I cry out. Help me to find joy in You, for Your joy will be my strength. May I sense Your presence in my hour of need.

In Jesus' name I pray. Amen.

Printed in Great Britain
by Amazon